*Praise for*

# BLOOD
# ORANGE
# NIGHT

"In this raw and captivating debut, journalist Bond chronicles her volatile descent into a benzodiazepine addiction. . . . Pairing her unsparing candor with the same deep compassion she finds in the physician who helped her level out, Bond's narrative casts a burning light onto the hazards of overprescribing and the threat it poses to vulnerable people. This cautionary tale stuns."

—*Publishers Weekly* (starred review)

"A harrowing memoir about a class of drugs as dangerous as opioids. . . . Bond's sharp critique of big pharma and the broken American health care system sounds an urgent alarm. A vivid chronicle of suffering."

—*Kirkus Reviews*

"Bond's story, with lines like 'the blood orange night turns red and screams through my eyes,' is an eloquent cautionary tale."

—*Booklist*

"A page-turner memoir chronicling a woman's accidental descent into prescription benzodiazepine dependence—and the life-threatening impacts of long-term use—that chills to the bone."

—*Nylon*

"Deeply personal insight into the ongoing benzodiazepine epidemic."

—*AV Club*

"An extraordinary memoir of an accidental addiction, and what it took to recover. . . . Propulsive and vivid."

—B&N Reads

"In her propulsive, poetic memoir, *Blood Orange Night*, Bond narrates her experience in harrowing detail. . . . Told with a journalist's commitment to fact and a poet's touch."

—*Shelf Awareness*

"An engaging testament to the powers of self-advocacy and resilience written with lyrical clarity and heart. This cautionary tale will help many understand how prescription drug dependency can happen and the strength and courage required to overcome it. Highly recommended."

—*Library Journal*

"There is a line in this evocative memoir that I will not forget, for it so perfectly sums up the effect that benzodiazepines have had on millions of lives: 'Benzos are the thief that steals everything you own a piece at a time.' In *Blood Orange Night*, Melissa Bond writes of the thief that crept into her life with the narrative skills of a fine novelist."

—Robert Whitaker, author of
*Anatomy of an Epidemic* and *Mad in America*

"*Blood Orange Night* is a beautifully written and exceptionally moving firsthand account of Melissa Bond's struggle with addiction to benzodiazepines. It should be read by anyone considering taking or prescribing medication for insomnia."

—Irving Kirsch, PhD, author of *The Emperor's New Drugs*

"A terrifying, fascinating story chronicled in a fever-dream of a book. Bond's words crackle with vulnerability and pain but also—as she climbs out of the darkness in which she has been living—hope, strength, and love."

—Eilene Zimmerman, author of *Smacked*

"*Blood Orange Night* made me feel all the feelings. Within the first few chapters, I laughed, cried, and got goosebumps. I cycled through sad and angry, followed by grateful and then outraged and sad again. I finally landed at hopeful. This book will make many feel understood and give them strength to fight the next fight. I loved it."

—Amy Lyle, author of *We're All a Mess, It's OK*

"Due to its incredible—and incredibly gripping—narrative, one would like *Blood Orange Night* to be fiction, or even science fiction. But this memoir tells a story that's too true: a physician prescribes drugs to his patient without informing her of their addictive nature. By the time she finds out she's hooked, we are too. Melissa Bond has shaped her story with a poet's zest for language, a humorist's sense of timing, and a mother's desire to spare others pain. This is an immensely important and inspiring book."

—Beth Ann Fennelly, author of *Heating & Cooling*

"Melissa Bond breaks necessary new ground in her astounding debut memoir, *Blood Orange Night*. A significant and essential contribution that further eliminates generations of tired stigma towards addiction and recovery. Her storytelling and literary genius read right into your heart—taking you to the nexus of heartbreaking despair—while putting resilience, self-love, and a tremendous amount of hope on full display."

—Ryan Hampton, national addiction recovery advocate
and bestselling author of *Unsettled* and *American Fix*

"In *Blood Orange Night*, Melissa Bond manages to capture multiple simultaneous truths: the frantic riptide of insomnia, depression, and drugs, as well as the buoyant, innocent loveliness of children. Which makes this book a powerful memoir about becoming a parent as much as it's also a breathless and harrowing detective story about benzodiazepine dependence."

—Catherine Newman, author of
*Catastrophic Happiness* and *How to Be a Person*

# BLOOD ORANGE NIGHT

*A Memoir of Insomnia,*
*Motherhood, and Benzos*

## MELISSA BOND

GALLERY BOOKS

NEW YORK   LONDON   TORONTO   SYDNEY   NEW DELHI

Gallery Books
An Imprint of Simon & Schuster, Inc.
1230 Avenue of the Americas
New York, NY 10020

First Gallery Books trade paperback edition June 2023

GALLERY BOOKS and colophon are registered trademarks
of Simon & Schuster, Inc.

*Blood Orange Night* was previously published with the subtitle
"My Journey to the Edge of Madness."

Certain names have been changed.

For information about special discounts for bulk purchases,
please contact Simon & Schuster Special Sales at 1-866-506-1949
or business@simonandschuster.com.

The Simon & Schuster Speakers Bureau can bring authors to your live event.
For more information or to book an event, contact the Simon & Schuster Speakers Bureau at
1-866-248-3049 or visit our website at www.simonspeakers.com.

*Interior design by Michelle Marchese*

Manufactured in the United States of America

10  9  8  7  6  5  4  3  2  1

The Library of Congress has cataloged the hardcover edition as follows:

Names: Bond, Melissa, author.
Title: Blood orange night : the true story of surviving benzodiazepine
    dependence / Melissa Bond.
Description: First Gallery Books hardcover edition. | New York : Gallery
    Books, 2022. |
Identifiers: LCCN 2021045637 (print) | LCCN 2021045638 (ebook) |
    ISBN 9781982188276 (hardcover) | ISBN 9781982188290 (ebook)
Subjects: LCSH: Bond, Melissa—Health. | Insomniacs—Biography. |
    Benzodiazepine abuse. | Insomnia—Psychological aspects.
Classification: LCC RC548 .B66 2022 (print) | LCC RC548 (ebook) |
    DDC 616.8/4982—dc23/eng/20211110
LC record available at https://lccn.loc.gov/2021045637
LC ebook record available at https://lccn.loc.gov/2021045638

ISBN 978-1-9821-8827-6
ISBN 978-1-9821-8828-3 (pbk)
ISBN 978-1-9821-8829-0 (ebook)

*To Jonny and Cash, under whose love and tutelage*
*I've become the kind of human I've always wanted to be.*

*And to all those who've suffered or are suffering under this crisis.*

In the midst of winter, I found there was, within me, an invincible summer.

—Albert Camus

Let everything happen to you: beauty and terror.

—Rainer Maria Rilke

may my heart always be open to little
birds who are the secrets of living

—E. E. Cummings

# CONTENTS

CONTENTS

# BLOOD ORANGE NIGHT

# PREFACE

WHEN I FIRST STARTED FALLING AND the bruises formed a map of yellows and browns on my body, I touched them and said, "This was my sway in the kitchen," "This was when I stumbled over the chair," "This was in the high grass outside, holding my daughter, Chloe." When I first started falling, I was blinded by a heavy fog of denial. It took a while for me to realize the insidious seep of drugs prescribed by my doctor for sleep were reducing me to nothing but bone and air. I was simply following my doctor's orders. I was in a free fall.

When my doctor initially gave me a prescription for Ativan, I knew nothing about it. Now I know it's a high-potency, fast-acting sedative hypnotic in the family of drugs called benzodiazepines, or benzos. Those in this family include Klonopin, Xanax, and Valium, among others. By the end of the 1960s, Valium was the top-selling psychotropic drug in the country. In the 1970s, it became the most widely prescribed drug of any kind. It was everywhere. Mike Brady popped a few on the television show *The Brady Bunch*. In the 1979 movie *Starting Over*, Burt Reynolds's character had a panic attack. When his brother asked, "Does anybody have a Valium?," every woman in the store opened her purse. Most memorable is the 1966 song written by the Rolling Stones, earning Valium the memorable and iconic name "mother's little helper."

In 1979, Senator Edward Kennedy held a Senate Health Subcommittee hearing on the perils of benzodiazepines, claiming they "produced a nightmare of dependence and addiction, both very difficult to treat and recover from." Shortly thereafter, *Vogue* magazine called the pills "a far worse addiction than heroin." Popularity dipped, but in the 1980s benzo popularity surged again after Xanax was brought to market as a treatment for those with panic disorder.

When I was prescribed Ativan in 2010, I didn't know the medical literature advised occasional use only, two to four weeks maximum. I had no idea long-term prescriptions were on the rise despite warnings of high addiction potential, or that overdoses and deaths from these drugs would soon rival those caused by opioids.

All I knew was I was a new mother with two infants, one with Down syndrome, and I wasn't sleeping. My marriage was faltering, and I was desperate to try to save it. I was desperate to care for my children without the constant struggle of feeling like an insomniac ghost. "Take these," my doctor told me. And so I did. Frantic for sleep, I took them month after month, my mouth wide-open like a hungry carp, trusting my doctor, who I believed knew what he was doing.

# PART ONE

## *Insomnia*

# ABC WANTS TO KNOW

*November–December 2013*

*First the light sinks to shadows; then the light is eaten.*
*Have you felt this? Have you been in this room?*
*What does one do with nights when there is no fleshy velvet of sleep?*
*It happened to me, quick as a shot and out of nowhere.*
*I don't know how many days it's been since I've slept. Two? Four?*

IT'S WINTER, AND SNOW IS HUNCHED like odd animals on the trees, when I receive the email from *ABC World News with Diane Sawyer*. One of the producers found my mama turned benzo withdrawal blogs. I'm amazed I've been able to write because of the sickness—the shivering of my eyes in their sockets, the muscles flickering like butterfly wings. Reading becomes impossible until I do the needed thing to beat the symptoms back. But still I write. I must. I don't need eyes to *tap*, *tap*, *tap* the black squares on the computer keyboard.

Sometimes I think if I can tell the story, I'll survive. Also, I'm pissed. For me—for others like me slipping into the dark. I try to write with technical and scientific accuracy to modulate my fury. I want people to understand this isn't anomalous. I cite the medical literature. It's all there, I say. Just look. There's a mountain of us who have been buried with this sickness; a continent. I don't know if this works. All I know is I've been writing about this thing that's happened and now ABC wants to talk to me.

The producer is from New York. Her name is Naria or Narnia and I imagine her with red hair, fiery and ready to dig in. "I found your blogs," she says. "We want to come to Salt Lake City to interview you." She asks if I'm willing to tell my story on national television. I pause. Jesus. Diane Sawyer. She's a legend, a high-ranking news journalist once suspected of being Deep Throat, the informant who leaked information to Bob Woodward in the Watergate scandal. When Diane became the first female correspondent on *60 Minutes*, I was in high school. I watched the show every Sunday on the floor of my mother's bedroom. The TV was stuffed at the end of my mom's bed and my brother and I had a six-foot swath of carpet on which to deposit ourselves for what we called "tube time." Watching Diane, I felt a doe-eyed feminist ardor I feel to this day.

My children are asleep downstairs.

My girl is three and my boy is four and I've had the sickness since before my girl was born. I don't know where my husband is, but I know he won't like it when I tell him they want me to be on national television. My sickness has taken him to the brink. I have no tumor to point to, no lab results over which we can cry together and show friends and family, no *known* story of what is happening to me. There is only the fire I tell him is in my head. There is the pain and my ribs poking out like railroad ties. He's tired and the fear has eclipsed him, turning everything between us to shadows. I don't blame him for this, but the wall between us aches. And now ABC. Now Diane Sawyer.

How can I say no?

When I was young, Diane interviewed Saddam Hussein and the Clintons. She got into North Korea when no one was allowed into North Korea. This woman has heft. She has moxie. Yes, yes, Diane.

My God! How can I even hold the fact they want to talk to me without melting into a wild but teary euphoria?

This story's tricky, and so much news has become a social narcotic. News as candy; news as sensational distraction. And it's this machine of sensationalism that has me nervous and uncertain in the face of Diane and her producers. I want to tell this Naria or Narnia that I'll consider being interviewed, but I won't prostitute my sickness to the media's love of McNugget news bites.

I'm cynical right now. It's part of the sickness. Forgive me.

My son makes his "hoo hoo" sound from his crib downstairs. His Down syndrome has made us all more tender than we could imagine. How will being on national television affect my family? How can I protect them? I must ask Narnia why they want to interview me. I will *not* agree to an interview if I'm to be their prime-time pity sandwich. Because this is so much more than *my* story. This is the story of millions of people just like me. I just happen to have survived. I just happen to be upright.

I write the producer, terrified.

Yes, I say. I'll do what I can.

# HIS HEART

*June–July 2008*

IT STARTED FOUR DAYS AGO. CONTRACTIONS through the night, starting and stopping. There's a palette of pain—dark, light, hollow blue, heavy blue, liquid red like fire. Sean and I were sure the baby would come easy. We'd prepared. I felt like an Amazonian. We'd taken birthing classes. When labor finally came, I breathed and breathed and first it was ten hours, then twenty, then thirty. Friends came and sang folk songs and played guitars for six hours before giving up and going home. Our doula banged a drum. Call the child out, find the rhythm that will seduce. We drove to the hospital, drove home. There was no sleep. Take black cohosh. Walk from the red rug of the living room to the wild greens growing in the backyard. Finally, at hour forty, we went back to the hospital and I was strapped in, measured, watched on a monitor that had a little stork flying across the screen to represent the baby's heart—which was failing.

At hour forty-eight, the room filled with a swarm of blue scrubs. I was on a bed with wheels and we rushed down the halls, ob-gyn trotting alongside. I saw the almond dust of hair on his upper lip. Sweat beaded and disappeared. In the room, I was anesthetized; a white whale beached on the shore in this lightblare room. Sean hovered. My boy was cut out. I smelled my flesh burning and then he wailed. His heart has continued to beat—my boy, arrived finally into the world.

And now, four days into our stay at the hospital, I'm drunk with sleep. The nurse opens the door. It's 2:00 a.m. She's a dark specter, her body backlit by the fluorescent hall lights.

I lurch up, electric. Something's wrong. "What is it?" I ask.

"It's Finch," she says. "We need to bring him to the neonatal intensive care unit right *now*. He's not getting enough oxygen."

I'm up and stumbling. I shake Sean, who's been asleep on the bright orange window seat that doubles as a bed. I'm hazy with Percocet, but my body knows something is very wrong.

I'm in my hospital gown with the wolf slippers Sean gave me. We'd thought they were hilarious when he brought them home months ago. They're huge wolf heads, twice the size of my feet. Clownish. Now they add a surreal element as we jog through the halls.

At the NICU, we scrub frantically using the special bristled brushes. We use a strong antibacterial soap and are directed to scrub up to our elbows. As we try to find the room Finch is in, Sean and I pass several unused incubators along one wall. They're the size of washing machines.

When we arrive, the nurses are putting a cannula up Finch's nose to deliver oxygen. Sean and I stand side by side, paralyzed. Finch cries at having the tubes shoved into his little nostrils, and with each howl there's a corresponding wail in my own body.

Nurse Robin explains that Finch will get oxygen. All his vitals will be monitored with excruciating detail. They're starting antibiotics right away. "The doctor will give the order, but they'll likely perform an EKG to check his heart," she says. We stay for hours, taking turns holding Finch. When we return to my room eight hours later, he's asleep on the warming slab, his little bird chest barely rising and falling under the thin blanket.

And now, on day five, we will leave and Finch will stay in the NICU.

In my room, the nurses begin the process of discharging me. Sean and I sign papers and take the little tote they give us that has pamphlets on breastfeeding and immunizations and a DVD called *Don't Hit, Take Time to Sit*, about how to avoid throttling your newborn. After gathering all my things, they tell us to go home and get some sleep.

"Come back at five," one of the nurses says. "They should have the results from the EKG back by then."

SEAN AND I conceived Finch less than two weeks after getting married. It was the kind of thing that steals the breath in mid-step. We'd been tangoing a lot post-wedding, as you can imagine, but the ultimate conception tango was just after our visit to Takashi, our favorite Salt Lake City hipster sushi joint. We'd started with the Volcano Roll. After that, we ordered buttery sablefish and the Red Hot Jazz. Waiters came and went, hovering next to our table, not wanting to interrupt. The restaurant evaporated around us. We were giddy with marriage and delicate sablefish and sake. So giddy, we danced a fierce tango in the car just outside Takashi. Then we went home and tangoed in the kitchen. Our steps were slow and breathless and heated, and when we made it to the bedroom, it was only to collapse into a warm marital heap. We were newlyweds and the world shimmered.

Just a few weeks earlier, when we'd discussed my going off birth control, I was sure my being thirty-eight years old would mean months or more before we'd have a taker of any kind. I told Sean that the lady in charge of pulling files in my brain circuitry would have to shuffle *way* back to get the information on what sperm was and how to use it. "Seriously," I said, looking as serious as I could, "she's old. She hasn't seen this file in decades. It'll take *forever*." This bit of rhetorical strategizing was entirely for my own benefit. Sean had told me two months into our courtship that he wanted kids. *Two months.* His biological clock was screaming. I, on the other hand, was sure my cosmic alignment would render me infertile at worst, difficult to knock up at best. Either way, I thought we had time. What we had was twelve days, give or take.

Sean and I had been married around three weeks when I got up from the kitchen table in the morning to drive to the grocery store. I didn't think. I drove. Once there, I bought a pregnancy test. I was being ridiculous—I knew it—but I couldn't help myself. There was just no *way* I could be pregnant. I kept saying this to myself while I drove and purchased and ran home to pee on a stick. I told myself this while I looked down at the little blue plus. I told myself I was silly, ridiculous, paranoid, while I peed on the second stick. And then I gawked. I sat in that bathroom for a long time staring at the walls. I'd been the baby of the family. I'd never babysat, never even changed a diaper. Married all of three weeks and I was suddenly, undeniably pregnant.

And though I felt unready, unsuited to motherhood and stunned with the suddenness of creating a human in my body, something happened when I got pregnant. I fell in. Motherhood is like this. Parenthood is like this, but women are given the mama cocktail that drinks us in and we become new creatures. I woke every morning and sat, hands around my cup of tea at our tiny kitchen table in our bungalow. "Take a picture of me," I'd tell Sean. And when I pulled my shirt up, he'd say, "Still looks like a beer belly," or "Today you're a small cantaloupe." And we'd marvel at how fast my body was changing.

AFTER DRIVING HOME from the hospital, Sean and I fall asleep. We jolt awake just in time to race to the hospital before the shift change at five o'clock. We jump into the car and I tell myself to focus on what's in front of me. Dashboard. Street signs. That same inane billboard for plastic surgery depicting three breasty melons of increasing size. The sky is the color of chalk, as if all texture has been erased. I feel my heart thumping in my chest. *Heart*, I think. No, not that—just look at the billboards.

At the NICU, we scrub vigorously. We walk fast, trying not to break into a jog. In room three, Finch is asleep, but the new nurse says we can pick him up if we want. We have to be careful of all the tubing and wires. I'm afraid of pulling something out. I tuck my hands under him and feel the warmth of his bundled body. He's so tiny, barely five pounds. I hold him against my chest. Sean stands up and walks around the little room. He sits. He looks at me and looks at the floor. We wait.

Finch's body is the size of half a loaf of Wonder Bread—so tiny, barely there. His hands are little fisted walnuts. I don't ever want to let go of this body—these eyes, this tiny belly. After ten minutes of holding Finch tight to my chest and pacing the small room, Dr. Templeman walks in. He's around fifty, with kind brown eyes. He feels nothing like the other doctors we've met in the hospital. He wears khakis and a button-down shirt and has the air of a monk. He settles into a chair in front of us and asks how we're doing. We don't know how we're doing, Sean tells him. We want to know about Finch's heart. We want to know our boy is okay. Dr. Templeman sighs. He looks at Sean and then me before leaning forward and placing his elbows on his knees. "The EKG came back," he says, "and Finch's heart is just fine." He pauses, his kind brown eyes looking into us. I feel air come back into my lungs. "But the blood work has also come back. Finch has tested positive for trisomy 21. He has Down syndrome."

All sound drains from the room. My throat locks up. My hands go numb against Finch's little body. Dr. Templeman sits across from Sean and me looking so full of compassion that I can only choke on the tears lodged in my throat. I can't cry or wail because the torrent of emotions floods me while my brain battles something that feels incomprehensible. I understand completely, but I don't understand at all. How can our beautiful, perfect Finch have Down syndrome? People with Down syndrome have always been strange to me. The ones I've seen always seem to wear Coke bottle glasses. They're heavy, with wide-set eyes. And they're retarded. The word suddenly becomes something new to me. Retarded. What does that mean, anyway? Slow? My boy will be slow? My boy may or may not talk? My mind races and slows, trying to find a place to land—something that will help me gain footing.

"How will we know how to take care of him?" I finally ask. And now I'm crying. I've never known anyone with Down syndrome. I've never even known anyone who's had a relative with Down syndrome.

At some point a Diane Arbus photo flashes in black and white in my mind. In 1970, Arbus traveled to upstate New York to photograph the people who lived in institutions for the mentally retarded. There were a lot of these institutions back then—warehouses where people who were deemed damaged or mentally deficient could be put away so as not to be a burden on family or society. In the photo that surfaces from my memory, a group of four or five adults stand at a distance, holding hands in a field. It's Halloween, so a few of them are wearing clown masks and sheets that billow around their exposed, pudgy legs. And there's something about the way they hold on to one another's hands—as if they're the only hands they have to hold on to in the world—that makes the scene bleak and horribly lonely. But this picture makes no sense to me as I look at my beautiful boy. I've never imagined the people in the photos as having parents. I've never considered what it must have been like for those parents to have been told their child was deficient or imperfect in any way. What was it like for them? What was it like for the children who got sent away? The thought brings a fresh choke of tears. I try to keep myself together but I'm falling apart piece by piece in this tiny glass-walled room.

After answering our questions about physical and occupational therapies, Dr. Templeman leaves. I sit holding Finch. I look into his unwavering blue eyes and try to connect my idea of Down syndrome to his perfect little body. And in the space of a moment, all the mental pictures I've had of those people in institutions who looked so lonely and sad and different fall away. The only thing that has oxygen to breathe is the love I have for my boy. The anguish of those pictures evaporates in the love that feels like it's breathing me. In and out, in and out. Nothing but love. And in this new context, everything shifts in how I feel about people who have Down syndrome or who have a different way of being in the world. I don't care that he has an extra chromosome. I don't know what it means or how we'll help him, but I know that we'll learn. I love him with a power that turns my tender heart liquid.

Sean and I stay into the evening. We go out for dinner and our young waiter seems to feel the crush in the air around us. After we finish eating, he brings us a massive piece of chocolate raspberry cake. "On the house," he says, his voice soft. "I just had a feeling you needed this tonight." I start to cry again. The simple kindnesses of Dr. Templeman and chocolate cake, together with my fear that I won't know how to care for Finch, bring an unstoppable flow of tears. Sean puts his hand over mine. He's crying too.

"Thank you," I say to our waiter, who's near tears himself.


IT'S NOT THAT night, but the next that I lie awake thinking of Beauty. In my twenties, I'd gone to one of those fancy liberal arts schools that emptied my pockets and filled my head with philosophies I would hold like glorious, ancient rocks. These philosophies had weight; they had heft. I returned to them often when I felt myself ungrounded, unmoored by any of the great confusions life could offer. I read Plato and Aristotle and Socrates. I studied Galen and Archimedes. I read the epics. All of them talked of Beauty and Virtue and Truth, and so many of them filled my head and my mouth. Sometimes it felt like I'd place those ancient rocks in my mouth and turn them over, placing my tongue here and there to feel for the sharp places and feel for what was right. Sometimes they were smooth and sometimes they cut my tongue, but I could always press myself against their solidness.

In those long nights without Finch, I think of Plotinus, the third-century philosopher and author of *The Enneads*. He described stars as letters inscribing themselves in the sky. He believed every moment was filled with signs and that the events of the world were coordinated, that "everything breathes together." I've loved this idea for a long time and give Plotinus a break for not knowing stars are a bunch of unbreathing, long-dead celestial matter. The image of the universe and all the things in it breathing together has long been a balm to my occasional bouts of cynicism and existential angst. I feel the Plotinus rock in my mouth. What would he say about Finch? How would he explain this beautiful boy's arrival in my universe? I feel a blind, burning love and wonder, *Is this Beauty? Is this kind of Beauty meant to cut one open at the seams?*

A day later, standing outside the hospital after visiting Finch, Sean and I make phone calls to our close circle of friends and family to tell them about Finch's diagnosis. I watch Sean pace in the hospital parking lot, the phone pressed against his ear. He calls his mom and sisters. I call my mom, my brother, my dear friend Ivy, with whom I share a love of writing, and a few other friends. It's awful only when the response is awful. The worst is a friend's awkward "I'm sorry," as if a mistake has been made, as if my boy himself is broken. I tell myself my friend doesn't know what to say, that perhaps his expression of regret is because of the difficulty of the situation, but the sting remains. And even worse is the knowledge that if the roles were reversed, I could have easily said the same thing. I could have fumbled, unconsciously adding loss to a tender heart that was trying to reassemble itself.

Sean and I scrub up before entering the NICU. We talk with Jerry, the speech therapist, at ten o'clock and Rachel, the occupational therapist, at eleven. We learn that a federally sponsored early intervention program will supplement physical and speech therapies until Finch turns three. Each conversation gives me more strength. The therapists hold us with their words and give us a vision of what it will be like to have a little boy who is different. He'll be the same, mostly. He'll do all the baby things, but they'll take more time. They will help us. We won't have to figure it out on our own. Their confidence and compassion give me the belief that I can do this. I can take care of my boy. The great mountain of fear that had risen in me begins to dissolve. We can do this. Our boy is so beautiful. And more than that, more than any of that, is the fact that we love him so completely. We're drunk on our love for him.

After lunch, we get the oxygen primer. Finch will go home with five tanks, twenty feet of tubing so we can walk around the house, and a monitor. The doctors tell us that lots of kids with Down syndrome have difficulty getting enough oxygen at first. They have no idea why. About 10 percent get sent home with the setup we've got. The cannula splits into two small tubes for his nose and is held in place via two very sticky circles of tape attached to his cheeks. Later that day, we walk out of the hospital a family of three, into the surreal landscape of the parking lot. The hospital was safe. Now we move under the shadows of the massive building, hefting tanks of oxygen and a little boy nestled in a car seat that looks like a battleship around his tiny body.

ON THE FIFTEENTH morning home, after giving Finch another bottle of the milk I pump with the industrial pump given to us by the hospital (hands-free using the specialized mama milking bra), Sean and I talk about writing an email to our broad community of friends. We've thought about it for days—how to phrase Finch's diagnosis. I want everyone to know he's healthy and different than we expected, and we love him. It feels simple to me. Sean's happy I have the words to write it. He feels overwhelmed, he says. The very fact that we have a baby has taken his heart on a journey, but Down syndrome has pushed that journey further than either of us could see. He wants to sit outside while I write the email. He wants to have another cup of coffee and not think about anything at all for a while.

I write draft after draft and everything sounds overly sentimental or wordy and I start feeling weepy again and have to stop. I look at Finch's sleeping face. How is it possible to love him so much so soon? I caress a small finger and he curls it around mine. After several minutes, I go back to the computer and start the email with his vital statistics:

*Finch Daniel was born June 26, 2008. He's five pounds, two ounces, bald as his papa, and has glacier-blue eyes that could stun an elephant. Many of you know he was diagnosed with Down syndrome. To us, this simply means he's more colors of the kaleidoscope than we could have imagined. We love him fiercely.*

# STING AND THE
# RADIANT BOY

*September 2008*

TWO AND A HALF MONTHS AFTER Finch is born, I return to my job as associate editor of the *Wasatch Journal*, a magazine serving the Intermountain West. I interview people like our governor, Jon Huntsman Jr., and other local celebrities. I work with smart and funny people, and the joy of being around adults who can get their own milk leaves me euphoric. I haven't realized how lonely being a mother to an infant can be. There's so much glorification of motherhood—all those media images of rosy-cheeked babes and their mothers staring beatifically into each other's eyes. Gerber propaganda. I tell my friends that somehow I must have missed getting the parenting manual I'm sure exists in some alternate universe that tells you the real nitty-gritty of parenting. The one that tells you you'll spend hours if not days speaking in monosyllables and watching the rain fall and not changing your milk-stained shirt just because no one will be there to see it and it will become milk-stained minutes after you change it anyway.

A friend of Sean's gives us the name of her part-time nanny, and now Christina, a Chilean immigrant and devout Mormon, watches

Finch gurgle on his baby mat for twelve hours a week. We settle into a routine. I write articles, go to the office, and work with writers for four hours, then return home to edit and help Finch do his physical therapy exercises on the U-shaped pillow that I fit under his chest three times a day.

TWO MONTHS AFTER Finch's birth, Sean and I go to see Sting. A friend has given us tickets and Christina promises to watch Finch until we get home. We're out-of-our-minds happy. For the past several weeks there's been a hushed uncertainty at work. My editor, Ivy, and I move quietly between our offices, sharing glances. I tell myself that the black waters of this Great Recession aren't lapping at our heels, but I know I'm lying to myself. I've taken additional assignments because our freelance budget has shrunk to a laughable amount. I interview Patrick Byrne, owner of Overstock.com. I write furiously, thinking that if we create something beautiful—so beautiful it will make people ache—the magazine won't die. Yesterday, in the kitchenette, Ivy said she hoped we'd at least get the winter issue out. I stared at the floor, mute. It's impossible to imagine the magazine failing. I just can't. So when Christina arrives at the house, giving us a night to indulge in a singer whose mark on the world is pure beauty, I practically cry.

"Don't forget to feed him at eight. He'll likely drink two bottles, so warm them at the same time, and if he doesn't fall asleep right away, play 'Over the Rainbow,'" I say. "And please pet the cat. Poor Goose isn't getting any attention at all," I add as she pushes us out the door.

"Go," she says in her beautiful, lilting accent. "We'll be fine."

And so we drive to USANA Amphitheatre, a massive outdoor concert venue with an amazing view of the mountains and, in the beer garden, painfully overpriced beer. Sean and I find our seats right in front of the stage and then Sean leaves to get a beer and mineral water. I wonder when the opening band will start. If they start in the next half hour, I reason, Sting will start in ninety minutes, give or take, which means we'll be home in maybe three and a half hours. I text Christina:

Me: *How's it goin'?*

Christina: *We r fine. He's doing his pushups.*

Me: *Does he miss me?*

Christina: *He's forgotten you exist.*

Me: *Thx.*

Christina: *Anytime.*

I turn off my phone and turn it on again. I'm being stupid. But I can't be sure a fire won't start somewhere in the vicinity of our house. If it does, or if Christina takes Finch out of the house and they're attacked by a rabid dog, I'll need my phone. I try to estimate exactly how long it will take Sean and me to get out of the parking lot and onto the freeway. Sean returns with our drinks.

"*Salud*," he says, raising a beer.

"*Salud*," I say, tapping his plastic cup.

The opening band runs onto the stage and a tsunami of sound crashes over us. I have no idea who this band is. I no longer know bands, which is crushing. Music has always been a mystical force to me. I've made more playlists than I can count and have loved knowing the best music able to capture deep wells of emotion. But in the space of just over a year I've left the archetype of hip young person and entered the archetype of mother. I pump my breasts with a machine. I eat standing at the fridge. When Sean and I were offered the tickets, I was euphoric to see Sting. Now I'm freaking out because I've left my child.

"Who's the band?" Sean mouths, nudging me with his beer hand.

"No idea," I mouth back.

He leans back and sips his beer. I watch a mid-twenties couple in front of me. The man cub wears black jeans predictably mid-ass with hiked-up white boxers. The girl is lanky, with silver hoop earrings and tattered black shorts. She has a tattoo running the length of her long calf. It's a stunning rendition of the elephant in Salvador Dalí's painting *Dream Caused by the Flight of a Bee Around a Pomegranate a Second Before Waking*—one of the Spanish surrealist painter's famous works. I lean forward as Lanky Girl looks around. I point to her leg and smile, giving her the thumbs-up.

"Cool," I mouth, smiling broadly at her to cover up the fact I've just given her the thumbs-up.

Sean and I watch the opening band and I look at my phone every five minutes to see if Christina has texted. She does not text that there is a fire.

When the opening band whose name I still don't know finally finishes their set, I tell Sean I'm going to get more drinks. Everyone standing in line seems to have either a tattoo or a piercing. I'm profoundly aware of the fact I'm wearing a maternity shirt. I have pads shoved into my bra so milk won't leak onto my shirt during the concert. I've never felt less sexy.

I leave the beer garden and walk between the upper and lower sections of the amphitheater. It's the same route I took to get to the beer garden, but on the way back I happen to look up at a section that's been cordoned off. I see a wheelchair pressed up against the iron railing. A young man sits in it. His smile is beyond radiant. He has wavy brown hair and deep-blue eyes trained expectantly on the stage. Next to him sits an older woman with silver hair. She has on a soft yellow sundress and one arm drapes over the arm of the wheelchair so she can hold his hand.

And then suddenly I see all of them. I stop in my tracks. There are bodies braced and wheeled, held fast with loving hands and belts running across their chests. There are some like Finch with wide-set eyes—like my boy, my beautiful boy. They're here, like me, to see Sting. A sign at the top railing says, SECTION FOR THOSE WITH DISABILITIES. My breath gets shallow and tears become little pools in the corners of my eyes. How did I miss seeing them on my way out? How could I have been so blind? It's then I realize I've been that kind of blind my whole life. An entire population, an entire segment of humanity, has been invisible to me. The Radiant Boy leaning forward with joy streaming out of him was invisible. His mother with the soft hands was invisible. My heart cracks open. Radiant Boy looks down at me. I put my mouth against my hand and kiss it, lifting it up to him. He doesn't lift an arm but smiles and kisses me back, pressing his lips into the air above me. *My God*, I think. *He's golden.* I go all at once into tears, my body slumping against the concrete wall. A minute later Sting is on the stage and I'm back with Sean. I'm up out of my seat, tears still wet on my face, singing at the top of my lungs.

THREE MONTHS LATER, Sean and I crush into a small wood booth at Cannella's, a local Italian restaurant, for the *Wasatch Journal*'s Christmas party. The recession tide has sluiced onto our shores, but we're defiant and drinking deep from the river of denial. *Hooray for us*, the party says. *We're not going to fold like those other magazines. Look at us having this great party with fat steaks and endless bottles of Petite Sirah. We're buoyant. We're huge!*

Our staff has grown thin in recent months as the publisher tries every angle to keep us alive. My colleagues join Sean and me in the dark booth. Sean tells a few lewd Santa jokes and soon someone chimes in about the difference between Tiger Woods and Santa (Santa stops with three hos) and we're all laughing. We talk over one another like crazed children until the restaurant closes. It's a lush Norman Rockwell moment. Hope and promise light us up, delightful and brilliant.

When Sean and I arrive home, he undresses me in our bedroom. We're all fingertips and mouths. Our bodies press hard together, tingling under the spell of the evening.

"Should we use anything?"

"No," Sean says. "You're breastfeeding. Shhhhh . . ."

Afterward, I curl against his warm back and listen to his breathing. *Just this*, I think. *Just this.*

# EASTER EGG BLUE

*February 2009*

I'VE BEEN PRETENDING IT DOESN'T MATTER, but once three weeks have gone by without a paycheck, I know it matters a lot. The *Wasatch Journal* is faltering, and our skeleton crew continues to thin. Staff are being laid off quietly, and each day I come in to find someone else missing. Our distribution manager is gone, then the graphic designer, then the copy editor. Those of us who are left have been promised a paycheck, but nothing has arrived.

Because Sean has his own landscape business, which is physically demanding, he likes to take winters off to recharge. He brings me coffee as I pull on my thermal underwear, sitting on the side of the bed to watch me dress, grabbing my ass like a seventeen-year-old when I bend over to retrieve my wool socks.

"You're going in?" Sean asks.

"Yes, I'm going in. Of course I'm going." I grab my keys.

"Is anyone going to be there?"

"I don't know," I say. "I hope so."

Prior to my job at the *Wasatch Journal*, I considered myself a guerrilla poet street scrapper, which I thought made my poverty sound more glamorous and intentional than it really was. In between poetry projects, I'd find paid work. I'd bend metal for metal artists and serve out-of-towners fancy beers on cork trays. I'd write divorce documents for lawyers. I'd turn myself into a graphic artist and design ads for high-end pet boutiques. I'd brave lockdown facilities for hardened addicts to teach writing. In between, I'd run poetry slams and organize flash mobs to recite verse on a street corner with everyone wearing pink hoop skirts. Guerrilla poetry. Scrapping. But always writing. Then I found magazines. Well, *a* magazine. One that I liked and that liked me, and we did a little dance and I was deliriously happy. I even had an official job title: Associate Editor and Poetry Editor. I had health insurance. I was the happy, humming girl. I was a glorious poet turned journalist singing the song of myself *and* getting paid.

I don't say anything to Sean, but I need this time in my office to remember who I am outside of the day-to-day minutiae of motherhood. I adore my son, but my work at the magazine gives the writer in me a room of her own. So I make the drive to the very white, very square building that houses the *Wasatch Journal*. I walk the two flights of stairs to our offices. The elevator has a handwritten "Out of Order" sign taped to the doors. It hasn't worked for weeks, and the entire building has the feeling of being hollowed out and on the verge of demolition. I'm fairly certain this is less about the recession and more about the fact the building appears to be managed by someone far away. I make up the story that the building is owned by a New York hedge fund broker looking for a place to store cash. They couldn't care less about ensuring the building is occupied, let alone whether the elevator works.

It's cold in the office. The heat was turned off several days ago, which is an undeniable death knell. But I still hope; I still sip from my cup of denial. I have four layers of clothing on and it's still cold. I heat a mug of water in the microwave that Ivy brought in from her house several weeks ago. There's no coffee or tea left in the kitchenette that sits off the main hallway. I riffle through papers at my desk. I have no windows. The walls in my office are a primer white, the kind of white that feels somehow both abrasive and dull. Someone long ago cut a square in the wall in front of me, right next to the door, and installed a piece of plexiglass. This plexiglass faux window allows me to look out onto the opposite wall, which is also white. It's 9:30 a.m. I sit at my desk, alone in this obscene whiteness with my mug of hot water and four layers of clothing.

After a half hour of staring muted at my computer, Ivy walks in, winks, and hands me my paycheck. The publisher has come through. Everything is fine and good, and I've been worrying needlessly. The Huntsman interview has been proofed and photographs have been supplied. Yes, there is a recession and, yes, magazines and newspapers are floundering like sad fish on a tide-stripped beach, but we will make it.

Two days later I'm home helping Finch with his little push-ups when Ivy calls. She asks me to eyeball the final proofs so we can send the magazine to the printers. I split my time between the office and home, which is damn lucky. I can pile toys around Finch and then edit on the couch until he breaks through the great wall of stuffed animals circling him. I consider his efforts to hurl the animals aside excellent therapy for his gross motor skills, but our cat, Goose, has become fearful of the occasional assault these stuffed animal circles represent.

"Can you get the proofs done by two?" Ivy asks.

"Yes," I say. "Two. No problem." This is the certainty I need. I feel strong and confident again. I'm making a living doing what I love, and I feel unstoppable. I effect a hip-shot nonchalance but inside I'm giddy. I imagine myself as the new Diane Sawyer poet rockin' the journalist beat with my own gonzo rhythm. I've been at the *Journal* a year and a half. Give me another year or two and I dream I'll get a toe in at *Rolling Stone* or the *New Yorker* or both. I'll meet Malcolm Gladwell for drinks and tell him how much his story about the radical technology of diapers changed my life. We'll become friends. Good God, life is glorious.

I decide to finish the proofs and then go to a yoga class. The energy in my body is like a tide. I need to move.

At two thirty, Sean takes Finch. We do the handoff and Sean kisses me.

"I'm glad you got paid," he says, reaching his hand under my shirt and whispering into my neck. "Maybe tonight we can celebrate."

EN ROUTE TO the yoga studio, free of the concerns for revolution or childcare, I make a right turn into the parking lot of our local grocery store. I hadn't planned this detour. I hadn't even thought about it until that very moment. But I get out of my car and walk in, making a beeline to the condom aisle. Ah, the condoms. The names alone are so very big, so Trojan in their pleasure. The condom aisle is where the home pregnancy tests are stocked, and I need one. No, I need two—better to buy two just in case. Because Sean and I haven't been using any of the aforementioned French letters. We haven't been using any kind of child deterrent whatsoever, and despite the fact I'm nursing *and* what's considered "geriatric" as far as motherhood goes, I feel a sudden, irrepressible urge to pee on a stick. I buy a two-for-one pregnancy test in a comforting pink box and, once in the car, roll the box up in my yoga mat.

Five minutes later I'm in the yoga studio, which smells of lavender and sweat. Shoes stack in neat namaste rows on the stairs. There's the happy hush I feel whenever I enter the yoga studio. I'm several minutes early and the bathroom that's always jammed with people trying to pee before getting into any kind of compromising position is open. I surge in, tucking my mat against me like a football.

The bathroom has a small shelving unit in front of the toilet with several rolls of toilet paper and a wood sign that says *Breathe* in white, painted cursive. I unroll my yoga mat and tear open the pregnancy test. My heart careens in my chest like a drunken toddler. *Breathe.* I pee on the first stick. I put the test on the shelf and wait, pants around my ankles. I stare at the stick as it turns blue. Easter egg blue. My God. It can't be. A slow buzz starts in my head. I tear open the second test and pee and wait. They aren't always accurate, these tests. You can have a false positive. But in seconds there it is: the blue plus. It's definite. Breath stalls in my chest. I have another passenger aboard.

I throw the test sticks into the garbage can and pile some toilet paper on top. I'm being ridiculous. I sign in with a big, shit-eating grin. People file in. Hushed tones fill the room. I spread my mat on the floor and lie down, trying to keep my shit together. *Keep your shit together! Jesus, this is a yoga studio.* The yoga teacher's name is Kim and she's lithe and beautiful. She sits on her mat in front of me as if she's sitting in front of a stream. And *lo! I am* the stream. And then we bow our heads and chant three oms. I start giggling uncontrollably. This is a problem of mine. Overwhelm of any kind sets off the giggles. It's an unfortunate coping mechanism, especially when in a yoga studio. I feel like a man having sex with someone for the first time and doing everything possible to distract himself and maintain the vigor of a stallion. *Imagine your mother-in-law! No, imagine a very, very sick kitten!* I start snorting, which is another unfortunate habit. I'm cracking up at the image of a sick kitten. I'm making little snorts into my mama bra tankini. *Death and carnage! Apocalypse! Zombies eating small children!*

I manage to get my euphoric shit together by the time we've moved from the stream and the oms to mountain pose. Still, I'm out of my mind. I'm ecstatic, looking under my arm while in down dog at the woman next to me and wanting to whisper in an embarrassingly loud voice—no, wanting to shout like a lunatic—"Hey, guess what? I'm pregnant! Can you fucking believe it?"

The next night I surprise Sean by asking Christina to babysit for a few hours so I can take him on a date to the Metropolitan, one of Salt Lake's swanky downtown restaurants. The Metropolitan advertised in the *Wasatch Journal* and, as payment, a few of us at the magazine got gift certificates. The Metropolitan is the kind of restaurant that has handsome Italian men waiting in the wings to fold your napkin into a quick swan when you get up to go to the bathroom. I feel both awkward and jubilant. It's such a silly thing, this kind of bourgeois napkin folding. But I've taken my man to the place of the fold, so we can sit next to the fire and order Bison Medallions with a Pomegranate Reduction and I can tell him I'm pregnant. *Again.* Earlier, I'd strolled into Planned Parenthood to take a *real* pregnancy test. The people at Planned Parenthood want me to plan well, and even though I've taken two home tests, which they assured me are fairly accurate, I wanted a third and final opinion. There's something about peeing into a cup in an office that feels more medically reliable than peeing onto a grocery store test at a yoga studio.

I wait for our bison to arrive before sliding Planned Parenthood's folded test results across to Sean. I sit on my hands, trying hard not to jump out of my seat and into the jaw of one of the hovering Italian men. Sean looks at the paper, then at me, then back at the paper as if it's something flammable.

"What's this?"

"Take a look."

"Uh . . . okay." Slow, unfolding of the paper. Eyes scanning the small print, confused. Finally, his eyes rise to the top of the sheet. He recognizes the name printed in boldface: Planned Parenthood.

"You went to Planned Parenthood?"

This is all going interminably slow. It feels almost scripted—the fumbling of the husband, the jittery glee of the wife. I'm out of my mind on baby hormones, and I recognize it—the evolutionary high in my body that has been turned on like a light switch.

"Yes," I say, cocking my head. "This morning."

Sean looks down again, but it's a wash. There are names of hormones with indecipherable numbers next to them running the length of the page. He looks up at me.

"You're pregnant?"

I nod.

"You're serious?"

"Yup."

He puts his hand on his forehead and starts rubbing it, fingers pressing in deep, as if somehow he can move the information in more quickly and have it make sense. We have a seven-and-a-half-month-old and I'm pregnant again. Hello, family.

"Wow," he says, rubbing. "Wow, wow, wow."

And then he looks up and smiles an awkward, vulnerable smile. It's the smile that felled me the moment I first laid eyes on him. My heart lurches.

"Wow," he says again. "You're pregnant. Oh my God."

After a few minutes and several gulps of wine, he stops rubbing his head and looks up, his eyes penetrating mine. "Have you told Finch?"

And then we fall into ridiculous, giddy laughter. The bison medallions have gotten cold, but we're in happy hysterics, unable to comprehend how this could have happened and then laughing at how much random sex we've actually been having—while Finch nods off in his seat in the living room; while he sleeps in the stroller we've parked next to the kitchen table; at midnight, at 5:00 a.m.; when it snows; when it doesn't snow. We laugh like two people at the edge of a cliff, ready to dive into water that shimmers at least thirty feet below us.

I CAN BARELY catch my breath at the suddenness, the corralling of everyone into the largest office, the one with the pretty but clichéd print of orange poppies in a field that someone had put up to combat the whiteness. I'd been so sure we'd make it. We'd sent the winter issue to the printers. We'd been paid. But this morning we're called in by the publisher's twentysomething son and are told that we're done, the *Wasatch Journal* is closed as of today, as of right now: Clear out your offices, take the microwave, there's just not enough money to keep us afloat. So sorry, and thanks, everyone, for your hard work. It's over.

# THE NIGHT RISES
# AND GROWS PALE

*February 2009*

IT'S BEEN TWO WEEKS SINCE THE *Wasatch Journal* closed, and I've been working to convince myself being unemployed is a positive thing. Jobs come and go, I tell myself. We're in a recession, and things die during a recession. I'm lucky the magazine lasted so long. I'll be a professional writer again someday, but for now I'll help Finch with his Down syndrome calisthenics. I'll perfect the gourmet casserole and work on my book while he naps. This unemployment will be a doorway, not a room with locked windows. It will be great.

It's still deep winter, so Sean has no work to occupy his days. He spends his time wrestling with light fixtures or huddled in his office downstairs, staring at the computer screen. He's been going out to the shed more and staying longer, returning with bloodshot, watery eyes. We agree I won't look for a new job, but still. He's suddenly responsible for all of us.

One morning in early February, I snuggle Finch into his high chair at the kitchen table. I'm trying to get him to eat a spoonful of mashed avocado when Sean makes the declaration that he's going to the mountains. He begins moving things around on the counter, looking under the little toaster oven and rummaging through drawers. He doesn't seem to notice my hand suspended in front of our boy's face. I make little hums as I nudge the spoon against Finch's lips.

I don't mind the time alone with Finch. I want a few hours to hustle up some work. I planned on pitching some women's magazines. There are few options nowadays, but the women's magazines pay well. I'll write about shoes or mama moxie. In the past week I tried some of my ideas out on Sean. "I could write about having a recession baby," I said, excited. "We need something." Sean's body got tense. Any mention of me taking time off to write seemed an intrusion, an unfair request for an extra heaping of our limited slices of time pie. He balked and reminded me that he works hard during the landscaping season hauling trucks of compost into suburban neighborhoods, digging trenches for irrigation and sod, and planting the precise number of irises and wild grasses. The work is exhausting, and he needs the winter to relax and have fun. I felt guilty and angry but swallowed all of it in the face of his furious dismissal.

"I can't find my keys," Sean says finally, lifting the bananas out of the fruit bowl.

"That sucks," I say. I tap the spoon against Finch's lower lip. "When's the last time you saw them?" Sean doesn't answer. He starts going through the drawer just under the fruit bowl. It's the catchall drawer, that repository for keys and broken pens and Post-it notes with the names and numbers of people we've forgotten entirely but can't bear to throw away. The keys must be there. He riffles through the drawer. They aren't there.

"I hate it when you move my shit. You're always moving my shit."

"What are you talking about?" I'm indignant. "And what's that supposed to mean, I *always* move your shit? I *never* move your shit."

My hand has been steadily pulsing against Finch's lips. When he opens his mouth, he gags against the baby spoon I suddenly thrust to the back of his throat.

"Oh, honey, I'm so sorry," I say. I wipe a smear of green off his cheek and ignore Sean. Both Sean's tone and the content of the accusation are hard—the kind of hard that renders me suddenly defensive, as if I've been caught red-handed huddled in the bathroom, smoking a joint, while Finch wails in the backyard. I take Finch into the living room.

"Papa can't find his keys," I whisper.

"Where are my *fucking* keys?" Sean yells.

After some tussling from the bedroom, during which I hear Sean moving his pile of clothes from one corner of the room to another, he goes silent. A minute later he's at the door, shrugging on his down jacket.

"Where were they?" I ask, trying to sound placid and not at all hurt. Or like throwing avocado in his face.

"They were in my windbreaker," Sean says. "Fuck, I'm late."

I'm SICK. ONE month into my pregnancy and my stomach is pinched as if in the jaws of a nutcracker. I remember this from my pregnancy with Finch. Nausea became the landscape that I lived in. It smelled of molding leaves and root rot and it ruined everything. There was nowhere to go, no amount of saltine crackers that could blunt its force.

Sean lies on the bed, reading a *New Yorker* magazine he's found under some T-shirts in his corner of the room. Snowfall has been thin and today is brutally cold, so he's stayed home from skiing to read and help with Finch. The magazine is open on his lap. It's dated June 2008, the month Finch was born. We find piles like this everywhere, ghosts of our pre-parenting days, reminders that we once had time to linger over books and articles, to have actual discussions. We were educated and thoughtful. We *read* things. We talked. Now almost all our discussions revolve around Finch's eating and sleeping. And shitting. This encompasses at least half of all discussions. Was today's shit peanut butter or curry paste? Was it watery or did it come out in those little nuggets that make him cry?

And now that I'm pregnant, there will be more of this. I wonder if we'll stop having sex or if we'll become parents whose conversations circulate around dinner and their children's bowel habits and recitals. We've been arguing a lot lately. Tension pulls at the corners of the house, as if the very rooms are growing smaller around us. I tell myself we're heavy with recession strain. We have a child with special needs, another one on the way, and no money coming in. Of course we're tense. But the tension is burrowing into my bones.

Finch is asleep in his bassinet. Sean doesn't look up when I get into bed. I trace my fingers up his thigh, hoping to pull him closer.

"Did you know Buckminster Fuller was expelled from Harvard?" he asks, still looking down at the magazine.

"No, I . . . is that the geodesic dome guy?"

"Yeah. He withdrew all his tuition money his freshman year so he could entertain a chorus girl."

"Seriously?"

"Yeah. They let him back in and then he got expelled again." Sean smiles to himself. He likes Buckminster Fuller. He keeps reading. My hand stalls. He looks up from the magazine.

"What?"

"*What* what?"

"You're staring at me."

"Oh. Um . . ." I fumble. I'm so painfully awkward with my need. "You know the poem I've been working on? 'Notes on a Pregnancy'? I was wondering if I could read it to you?" I recently wrote a list poem with forty lines to reflect the forty weeks of being pregnant. And I know it's nothing I can sell. It will not make me a famous writer and it will not buy milk, but, damn, it came like wildfire and I love it. I want my husband to love it.

"Sure," Sean says, sighing. He keeps the magazine open in front of him. His "Sure" is rigid. It's not the casual *Yeah, baby, that sounds great* kind of "Sure" but more of a *Let's get this over with as soon as possible* kind of "Sure." Maybe, I think, he really wants to hear the poem, but he also wants to read more about Buckminster Fuller. After all, it has taken him eight months to get to this issue of the *New Yorker*. He's conflicted, I tell myself. He's conflicted and stoned. He loves that I'm a writer, even if I'm no longer a writer who makes money. My husband wants to hear everything I write, especially poems about him and our new child. I'm being self-conscious, ridiculous. It's the pregnancy, the constant pulse of nausea. I'll read him the poem and he'll feel his heart surge and Buckminster Fuller will slide off our bed and we'll have amazing sex.

Sean pauses for a minute after I finish reading. "Huh," he says. He stares unblinking and my hand falls off his leg. The magazine is still open on his chest. He looks at me, then looks down, fingering the magazine. "Um. Thanks. You know—for sharing." Blank and cold.

SEVERAL NIGHTS AFTER reading Sean my poem, something rips me from sleep. Sean and I got into bed at 9:30 p.m. as usual. Finch was asleep in his little bassinet, his eight-month-old body still so tiny. I'd run one finger over the top of his velvety head before kissing him and turning out the light. Sean was out in minutes, one long leg thrown over mine, his breath deep and even. I drifted off. There was no dream. There was only the sweet lull of sleep and darkness and then the feeling of something smashing me in the chest.

I lurch up, gasping. Was there a noise? My heart slams, wild and unfocused. I freeze, listening. There must have been a noise. There have been so many break-ins on this street—the house next door, the one three doors down. I hold my breath. Slow rustling from the bassinet. A car driving by. Nothing more.

I get up and walk to the front room. Shadows move on the sage-colored walls. The big front window looks out onto the street and shows nothing but a tree backlit by the full moon. It's early spring but

I can still see little crusts of snow on the ground. I scan the darkness. Nothing. And still my heart tries to hurl itself out of my chest. I sit on the couch and stare at the walls, the shadows. *Maybe it's the full moon*, I think. *Maybe that's what's happening.*

Two hours later, I stand. I've described the house to friends as a small train car with two levels. "It's got the absolute *worst* feng shui," I've said, "but the backyard is amazing." The front door opens right onto a street of cracked and wounded pavement. Inside the front door, a small room with a window looking out onto the street serves as our living room. The living room narrows to a hallway that goes to the kitchen. Sean's and my bedroom juts off the hallway like a little side cabin. The tiny yellow kitchen is the last room before the hall stops at the back door and the stairs that lead down, back under the kitchen, to the basement. Our single bathroom is tucked away near the back door and shares a wall with the kitchen. We are a train car with adjacent cabins. The carpeted basement runs the length of the house, ending in a small boxed bedroom with a single window that looks up at the cracked pavement outside. The entire house from top to bottom is maybe one thousand square feet.

I WALK FROM the living room, through the hallway, and into the bathroom. I put my hands on the sink, leaning against the porcelain. I splash cold water on my face. People do this kind of thing in movies all the time: hands on the sink, looking into the mirror. Minutes pass. I take quiet gulps of air, waiting. The water doesn't help. I walk out of the bathroom and back to the couch. Small waves of nausea are cut with a feeling that my arms and chest are threaded with electricity. I check the window again. Hours pass. I tell myself that a night of missed sleep has everything to do with the pregnancy. There have been stranger things. *Wait it out. Sleep will come. Sleep has always come.*

When dawn breaks, I haven't slept. All I can do all day is watch Finch practice his Down syndrome calisthenics until he cries and then falls asleep. That night Sean comes home and makes some kind of chicken and I eat it. I'm beyond relieved when night arrives. I imagine that we will put Finch to bed and we will turn out the light and I will crash like I've never crashed before.

But I don't crash. Two more nights and days pass and I don't sleep. I meditate, tell myself to be present and just rest. The digital numbers on the clock blink by: 12:00 a.m.; 2:32 a.m.; 3:17 a.m.; 4:00 a.m.; 6:12 a.m. The clock becomes an obsession, the light outside changing from ink to smudged charcoal. I do lunges through the hallway to exhaust my legs. I do squats by the back door until my body burns. Maybe I sleep one night. I don't remember looking at the clock between four and five. Maybe I get an hour. Maybe I get thirty minutes or ten or twelve. I walk through the house and sit and walk again. Maybe I slept. *My God, what's happening?* I'm a wounded animal, soft and hunched over. I want to bang my head against the wall out of terror that it will happen again, that it will never end and I'll go psychotic and have this feeling of glass in my body forever. I decide to try NyQuil or a bunch of whiskey. *I'll drink both. No, I can't drink NyQuil or whiskey. I'm pregnant.* Jesus.

In the mornings Finch makes his early-morning squawks. I walk downstairs, to the crib we've set up for him in the basement hallway that now serves as his baby room. I bring him to the bedroom and lay him next to Sean. I make coffee. *I'll sleep tonight,* I think. *This is crazy. The body can't live on so little sleep.* My God, I miss having someone to help, even for just a handful of hours a week. We cut Christina's hours when I lost my job at the *Journal*. I knew it was a risk and it was only a matter of time before she got a full-time job. She introduced us to her sister Josefa, but Josefa was erratic and had classes at the community college that made scheduling difficult. Besides, I could tell she didn't like watching Finch very much. The few times we had her come over, I'd come back after doing a few errands to find her glazed in front of her iPhone, Finch rolling in the deep amid the heap of stuffed toys.

I tell myself I can make it through by pretending the day is made of a series of small stones. One step, two steps. I only have to do one at a time. Thinking of the day in these parceled-out pieces makes it bearable. If I imagine taking care of Finch for twelve solid hours with snow hanging in the clouds and no sleep, I feel like I'm going to completely lose it.

THREE DAYS AND nights pass. I become a woman on fire. My head burns. My arms and legs burn.

"I didn't sleep again last night," I say to Sean over breakfast, jostling Finch on my lap. "Maybe an hour."

"It just feels like that," Sean says, throwing his hand out loosely as if brushing the insomnia away like a bit of hovering lint. "You had to have slept more."

"I don't think so." I try to be both honest and strong but I'm desperate for him to react with worry, to call the doctor friend he met at Ultimate Frisbee, to hit a bright red button of high alert so I can fold over and let myself fall apart. But he's guarded, his body rigid in the cold kitchen.

"Maybe you can sleep this afternoon. When Finch naps."

"Yes, maybe. I don't know."

"There has to be something . . ." Sean trails off, picking up the frying pan. "Can I make you some eggs?"

Two more nights pass. I'm losing my sense of time. Every morning Sean gets up and I make coffee and every day we pretend this isn't happening. He leaves to do some errands and I steel myself. One morning I sob with Finch on the bed. I forgot where I'd put him, forgot where my child was sleeping, and ran to each room looking for the little movable rocker with the dangling hippos and elephants that I know I'd laid him in and put down somewhere. When I found him in his bassinet, he gazed up at me with calm blue eyes and I hunched over him, bawling, holding his happy little foot in my hand.

When I tell Ivy about the insomnia, she wonders if I am perseverating, turning some unhappy stone over and over in my mind until all hours, but it isn't true. My mom calls on occasion and offers the same explanation. I lean my head against the phone, crying. "You must be worried," she tells me. "Honey, anxiety will kill your sleep." Every night I curl on the couch and try to meditate. I search "hypnosis for sleep" on the computer and listen to a man with a lisp tell me I'm drifting in purple clouds. Nothing works. All I can think all night is: *I'm not sleeping. I'm in a purple cloud and I'm still not fucking sleeping.*

Days with Finch are a torture. He wails for me to pick him up, wails for me to put him down. I follow the motherhood routine, feeding him yams and beans, keeping my voice high and lifted, changing his diaper at two-hour intervals because I won't remember otherwise. What does one do with an infant boy all day? I take him for drives up Emigration Canyon. Just strap him in and drive. Something terrible is happening. It's been over a week, and now, when I sit, my arms and legs make little jerks like they're covered with flies. I have to concentrate on the smallest task. How many tablespoons for a pot of coffee? Has Finch eaten? Has he slept?

My growing sleep deprivation is an abstraction to Sean. He hardens around its terrifying uncertainty, taking Finch when he gets home so I can lie on the bed and stare at the white walls. We get into bed at night and Sean slips so easily into sleep. I wait until his breath deepens before getting up and taking my place on the couch. In the morning he sees my bleary face.

"Did you sleep?"

"An hour," I tell him.

"You must have gotten more than that," he says.

I begin registering things at half speed. One day I sit motionless at a green light until a man behind me leans hard on his horn. I imagine people asking me simple questions. I know there will be a gap before I answer. I haven't slept more than an hour a night for over a week. Maybe less than that.

During the night, I sit on the couch and breathe in, breathe out. The idea of an "I" has become a swinging door. I listen to the lisping man with my headphones plugged into the computer. My arms jerk as my body drifts and jerks up again. I research Aristotle and insomnia. I've always loved Aristotle. The guy was an intellectual Buddha and planted questions about virtue and ethics that have grown in me throughout my life. He spoke a lot about happiness as the prime mover for humans. He talked about balance and ethics and what it means to live a fulfilling life. I so often turn to the philosophers or poets when nothing else makes sense, but Aristotle's "On Sleep and Sleeplessness" is no help whatsoever. Aristotle was not an exhausted mother. I can't fault him for this, but his musings can only go so far for me. Even the German philosopher Nietzsche, echoing Clement of Alexandria, wrote that "the need of sleep is not in the soul." I bite my nails to bleeding without knowing it. *Entitled German bastard*, I think. *This body is a wasteland, Nietzsche, a beast dragged behind an endless burning light. You don't know what the fuck you're talking about.* I close the computer. Where's my philosopher mother? Where's the woman who digs deep into what it means to be human when you're also wrecked? I feel like a body under a train, ground down to nothing by lack of sleep. My eyes slip to the back of my head, eyelids fluttering closed and then shocked open by what? I don't know. Back to the couch, the bathroom, the cool linoleum of the kitchen. There's nothing to do, nothing but a persistent hum of bees under my skin and the feeling that I'm losing my mind.

After two weeks of the night rising and growing pale, Sean's tight hold on the fear of what's happening to me erupts. He finds me on the back-porch swing at 3:00 a.m. and finally understands that something in me is cracking. Night feels like doom now, the dark pulsing and alien. I sit on the swing and pound my head against his chest, begging him to just take me out.

"Come to bed," he says. "Please." He is frantic. If I lie in bed, surely I'd sleep. If he could feel my body quiet next to his, everything would be okay.

I begin making the rounds. I see a naturopath, a nurse-midwife, a sleep clinic doctor, a therapist, and a shaman. I tell them I can sleep only two hours a night. No, I say, sometimes it's three. Not often. I don't like medication, I say. I'm pregnant. But I'm desperate. Something is off. Some timing belt needs to be fixed. I figure one of them will know what's happening to my body. But they all essentially tell me the same thing: nothing can be done.

Each asked if I watched TV before bedtime. *No.* Vigorous activity? *No.* Overconsumption of vodka or hot chilies? *No.* And the inevitable question: Am I scared of having another Down syndrome child? A storm gathers inside of me. *No. No! No!!! Fuck you! Fuck all of you! How could you imagine my boy that way?*

Naturopath: "I'm afraid you can't take herbs because you're in your first trimester. You can't take much of anything, really. Try sitting with your legs up a wall and breathing through your left nostril for eleven minutes every two hours or so. It soothes the parasympathetic nervous system. Chamomile tea is good. We should look at some adrenal supplements. You sure you don't watch TV?" I do this for a week. Every ninety minutes, legs up the wall, finger clamped against the right nostril to enable left nostril breathing. It's a snotty business and not in the least relaxing. My parasympathetic nervous system is nonplussed. I do not sleep.

Nurse-midwife: "Unfortunately, you can't take sleep medication because you're in your first trimester. We don't want the baby born with no arms or legs, do we? Little torso of a baby? Try Benadryl. And earplugs work wonders. Keep up the good sleep hygiene."

Sleep clinic doc: "You don't have sleep apnea and that's all I can figure. We'd offer medication but you're in your first trimester. And, honestly, there's not much research that's done on pregnant women. Have you tried painting? Creativity can be a wonderful balm to the sleepless."

Therapist: "How do you feel about your son? Are you sure you're not concerned about having another child with special needs? No? Anxiety can manifest in a number of ways. And you may have PTSD from your C-section. I'd recommend meds, but you're in your first trimester. And you recently became unemployed, is that correct?"

Shaman: "You're in the belly of the big snake. Now I'm gonna blow some tobacco smoke around your face and bang on a turtle shell."

AFTER EIGHT WEEKS, my hands begin to shake. There's the feeling of being broken, of the head and body not being connected. Some puppeteer jangles my legs, my head. I wobble and crash into the kitchen, the bathroom.

Sean and I argue about whether to have the test to see if my growing baby has the normal number of chromosomes. The test is called chorionic villus sampling (CVS) and has to be done between the tenth and twelfth weeks of pregnancy. A huge needle will be inserted through my stomach and into the placenta. A doctor will wiggle and scrape with the needle so we can gather enough genetic material to know. A lab somewhere will analyze said placenta cells. They will tell us boy or girl. They will tell us if there is a surprise third chromosome. Sean and I argue about what to do if the test shows an extra chromosome.

"I don't want to know," Sean says. We're in the kitchen after dinner. Plates sit ignored in the sink while Finch sleeps on Sean's chest. "I don't see why you have to have the test. Can you imagine our lives without this little guy?" He strokes Finch's cheek.

I sigh. "Of course not, but . . . honey, some extra chromosomes are lethal." I'm trying to reason. I always try to reason around things in which there is no inherent reason. Like chromosomes. Like what you will do if they aren't all there or if there are more than are optimal. Like unexplained, pathological insomnia. I close my eyes. An electric sensation moves in my arms and legs. I force my eyes open.

"Listen . . . sweetie . . ." My voice cracks from exhaustion and the effort it takes to manage my fear about whether to have this test. "They can have a cleft that goes from the palate all the way up through the brain. They can have a defect where their spinal cord and all the blood vessels and everything poke right out of their back." Sean looks down at Finch. He doesn't look up. I wait. He starts to fiddle with Finch's fingers. I try again. "Remember the woman we met who told us her son had been born *without an asshole*? He had to have ten operations before he was two. *Ten.* The kid had a million-dollar asshole. We don't have the money for a million-dollar asshole."

"Yeah, okay," Sean says, his eyes flicking up. "You've made your point."

"Okay . . . *and*?"

"Yes, have the test."

"Well, I . . . I want you to be there. I'm going to have a foot-long needle inserted into my body."

"Okay. I'll be there."

"Okay."

We lapse into a silence vibrating with tension. We are a shivering, mile-long band of the unsaid. I force the burn of insomnia away and try to focus. I've been sleeping an hour or two a night for a month now. I can barely manage my own emotions, much less Sean's. Our silence is so heavy, and it says everything. We haven't gotten to the real point, the point of contention, the point that feels impossible to address because even getting close feels like it could draw blood.

"Okay," I say again, feeling like a monster for forcing the issue. "Listen, we're not making any decisions here, okay? I just want to know. I mean, my God, don't you at least want to *know*?"

Sean runs his fingers over Finch's sleeping face. "I just can't imagine making a decision if there's some kind of a problem," he says.

And the truth is, neither can I. It's the worst thing possible. And how will we even begin to decide what's considered a *problem*? There are the easy *This child won't survive outside of the womb* problems. But what about the *survival with complications* problems? What if they tell us we'll have a healthy but strangely built torso of a baby? What then? What's the point at which we decide this baby should be taken out of the system—*Whoops, bad timing, sweetie. Let's try again?*

The thing we can't bring ourselves to ask each other is what we'll do if our new baby has Down syndrome. I tell myself we won't abort unless there are severe medical issues. But genetic tests don't always catch these things. We won't know, for instance, if the baby will be born without an asshole until far into the game, if at all. Thinking about this gray area makes me sick. Going in willfully blind is worse, I tell myself. Much worse. We could compromise our ability to take care of Finch. We could end up living like so many hospital parents—going to support groups and telling ourselves that our child is a trouper and hovering at the threshold of each night, wondering if our child will survive until the morning. No, I am going to have this awful test. We'll address whether to play God when they call us with the results.

The test takes three days to process. Sean goes skiing with Finch towed behind in a cozy ski stroller and I'm alone when the hospital calls. The nurse at the end of the line clears her throat before giving me the potentially devastating news but she's finefinefine—a girl! My God, a girl! And she has absolutely normal genetic markers, the nurse says—no cleft palate, no neural tube defects, no small skull. I call Sean right away, jumping up and down with the phone in my hand, the fist of fear in my chest gone and my heart suddenly, for the first time in months, skipping down the street. We're going to have a girl and Finch will have a sister. She's a beautiful little seahorse in my sleepless ocean and I hold on to this fact like a buoy that's been thrown from a golden ship with everyone smiling and waving. In that moment, the insomnia burn in my body feels worth it. The black-dog hallucinations and the night fear wash away and for a few tender hours the world feels sweet and unburdened and full of light.

# SCRIBBLES ON A PAGE

*Late April 2009*

I'M WEAVING AS I WALK THROUGH the parking lot of the Intermountain Medical Center. I hold Finch in his portable car seat and focus on walking a straight line. Sean has started his landscape season in earnest and is hustling to rake leaves and prune trees for families far from here. I've been pregnant twelve weeks and the insomnia has become so severe, I'm under the impression I may be teetering near psychosis. An article on the website Frontiers in Psychiatry states sleep deprivation can cause "perceptual changes, including visual distortions (i.e., metamorphopsias), illusions, somatosensory changes and, in some cases, frank hallucinations." I know that on January 10, 2004, CIA general counsel Scott Muller suggested reducing the threshold of sleep deprivation from seventy-two to forty-eight hours. Anything over forty-eight hours was deemed "enhanced interrogation techniques," and a lot of people pretty much thought this was akin to torture and totally uncool. After days without sleep, people can become disoriented. Judgment is impaired. They may say nasty things to the person inflicting the sleep deprivation or maybe even their spouse. They may, in fact, feel some degree of hatred toward their spouse for no good reason at all. Hallucinations can set in after a day or two. The CIA does not have me in a room with my arms suspended above my head, but if they asked me something right now, I'd say anything. Anything to sleep. Kim Jong-un? Oh, yeah, I know the guy. Great hair. Kind of chesty, though, you know, in that chest bumpy kind of way. Me and Jong-un, we're tight.

My arms and legs burn like a light acid has been rubbed into my skin. The sun's way too bright, even with my dark sunglasses. Every sound, even the scrape of my shoes against the pavement, is a *boom!*, sonic and crushing. I twitch with the effort of making it to the office of my nurse-midwife. I weave. I see shadows of people where there are no people. I see cars backing out when nothing is moving. *Just get to the office*, I think. *They'll help. Don't let go of the handle to the car seat. Don't forget Finch on the burning pavement after you've set him down so you can rest against someone's big white truck.* Everyone has big white trucks in Utah—something about the landscape, the great expanses of mountain and sky. They need a vehicle that takes up space.

I make it into the cool, controlled climate of the hospital. The lobby is sharp and clean and white. The elevator doors have a bright aluminum sheen that is so smudge-free, it must have its own staff of cleaners hovering in the alcoves, ready to rush in and buff the doors for thirty furious seconds after anyone enters or exits. I use the sanitary hand cleanser that's in increments of twenty feet throughout the hospital. In the elevator, I look down. I still have Finch. *Good*, I think. *Good. I haven't left him on the pavement. We're almost there.*

At the nurse-midwives' office, I stand vaguely at the check-in counter, waiting, staring into the air in front of me. I've brought milk. I've brought Finch's tiny squeaking alligator. I hover it over his head like a helicopter.

Two young girls make up the office staff. They swivel in their black office chairs, phones pressed to their ears. They look down and away from the air I occupy. They're busy. They're setting appointments and reminding women to take their prenatal vitamins. I wait. After ten minutes standing in front of them without acknowledgment, I give them my name and they direct me to the waiting area. I'm too tired to read the *Good Housekeeping* magazines on the coffee table. I don't look at any of the other mothers. I set Finch and his car seat on the carpet. I dangle the squeaking alligator.

After an impossible amount of time, a young girl in mauve scrubs opens the door to a labyrinth of offices. I'm ushered in. The girl has an acned chin and sensible shoes. She asks how I'm doing. I try to say something inconsequential, something to keep me from crying, something to deflect. This girl's job is to weigh me and escort me down the hall, nothing more. "Look at my son," I say. "He's going to crawl any minute now. He's going to steal my keys and crawl out of here and drive to a burger joint. Just watch." She laughs. I pretend to laugh. Ha ha ha. Life is funny, isn't it? Life is so funny. I'm on top of the world.

I sit in my room. It's unbelievably bright. Why do they make these rooms so bright? I jiggle Finch's car seat with my foot. He sees something in the air and gets this startled look, blue eyes growing big as headlights. I'm used to this look. Sean and I call it the "rapturous air" look. Finch gets all shivery and euphoric, as if William Blake himself has appeared, opening his hand to show Finch the face of God.

The nurse-midwife who walks in is not *my* nurse-midwife. This isn't Angela, the one who spent over a year in Guatemala teaching rural women how to deal with breech babies and hemorrhages and preemies. This isn't Angela, who sat with me in the hospital after I thought my water had broken early with Finch and told me that, no, all that extra fluid wasn't amniotic fluid but semen. This isn't Angela, who leaned in and whispered that perhaps my man was a wild boar, the kind known for producing over half a pint of semen at a time. Oh, we had a good laugh, me and Angela. She was damn funny. And smart. But this wide, nervous woman isn't my Angela. This is Mary Beth or Mary Ann, whom I've never met before this very moment. Angela is delivering a baby, I'm told. She's busy. She's hands-deep, and Mary Ann or Mary Whoever is taking her shift. She sits down to open my file in the computer and asks the one question, the awful question, that's a tiny prick against my membrane, pulsing with hemorrhage.

"So your weight's a little low. How are you feeling?"

Mary's soft white hands pause over the computer keyboard. She has a thin silver chain on her right wrist that catches in the crease of the flesh between wrist and arm. It's a pale arm. This Mary is pale. She's squinting at my record on the screen. Her mouth moves as she reads: *late-stage mothering, infant with Down syndrome, persistent insomnia.* Her mouth blows an escaped curl of brown hair dangling over her lips. *Insomnia. Persistent.* The curl has a practiced tousle that has been constructed with much hot iron curling. She has curled and arrived to take her shift at the nurse-midwives' office at the Intermountain Medical Center and she is now staring expectantly at me with that practiced nurse wait, calm but intense—an active waiting. She raises her hands higher above the keyboard. "Hmmm? Doing okay? Nausea?"

"I haven't been sleeping," I say, the blood beginning to gather in my face.

"Oh?"

"At all. I mean, some. But hardly." I swallow. I rock Finch's car seat with my foot.

"It's not unusual to—"

"I know it's not unusual. Occasional sleeplessness isn't unusual when you've got a baby. But what I'm having is not *occasional*." My emphasis on this word is hot. I can feel the word whip out of me as I glance at Mary. I've been told by friends and lovers that my eyes are "intense." I've always felt they were plain hazel eyes shaped like little almonds, but in my head they're unnerving.

"I'm sorry?" Mary has taken an inbreath and hasn't exhaled. Her hands remain suspended over her keyboard.

I keep talking and it's a slow fall down a steep staircase. There's an initial sense of being off-balance, the foot hanging out lopsided, the hands whirling in the air. And then there's the fall. I'm outside of myself looking in. I'm telling this Mary Whoever that I haven't done it, of course, I've only thought about it, but if sleep doesn't come, I may do something drastic. Clearly, this is something I shouldn't be saying. This is something that shouldn't be said unless one desires a sudden and swift psychiatric evaluation, but I'm saying it.

"Listen, Mary Ann or Mary Beth, I'm not sleeping. I've spent the past two weeks going to everyone under the sun and they've all told me they can't do anything. My son, Mary—I hallucinate when I watch him. Imagine watching your child and hallucinating dogs or people breaking into your house because you haven't slept." I pause, knowing I'm going to take it too far, knowing I should stop, but there's nothing left to do. My voice warbles, high and tight like someone stumbling at the edge of a cliff.

I wonder what kind of force it would take to really knock myself out. Even if I ran straight at a cinder block wall at full speed, I probably wouldn't have the requisite force. I'd just give myself a hard knock and the whole business would hurt like a motherfucker. I'd tumble over sideways into the weeds that would most definitely be there and I'd be awake amid the weeds and the trash with a stupid crush of blood in my hair. Then what? I begin crying.

I stare at a print on the wall of a young woman in a garden. The whole thing is in various shades of cream and the woman's hair is soft around her face. She looks well rested. She has a basket with violets on her arm and is bending over to pick more.

I look up at Mary Ann or Mary Whoever and wipe my eyes. I nod at the print. "Pretty picture," I say. She looks at me, looks at the picture and then back at me. It's clear this Mary hasn't been trained for such encounters. She's never dealt with someone whose cheese is sliding off the cracker. She stands and puts both hands in front of her as if to stop an oncoming train.

"I'm going to go consult with one of our doctors," she says, backing out of the room, hands still up like little fans. "Just wait here."

Clearly, something needs to happen. Something big. Mary Who-ever is going to call the big guns and pray. She will get down on her knees and pray in the little supply closet and I will begin crying again. I will keep crying even after she's exited the room. After several minutes Mary Whoever comes back in.

"We're getting you a prescription for Ambien CR," she says. "It's safe for the baby. You can also take two capsules of Benadryl. That will boost things." Mary is worried I will break down again. She's worried I won't get back up. And I'm worried that I'll break down and never come back. I can barely contain the fear that I'll never sleep again and will crumble into a blinding psychosis. It's the third week of an interminable April and I will take the little pills, because I'm terrified. I want to care for my son, but my body has never failed me in this way, never turned a sudden corner and skidded out in the horrific slow-motion skid that always seems to happen before a fatal and inevitable crash.

PART TWO

*The Book of Sleep*

# MANIC

*May 2009*

THE DAY I GET THE AMBIEN CR from Mary Whoever, I race home
with Finch. It is solved. Whatever was stealing my sleep will be remedied and I will be myself again, ebullient and ready for this new chapter. And that first night is a dream. I am out for seven hours—seven!
It is staggering. I feel so capable, my maternal strength so oxen. Oh,
ho—could I ever casserole now! I could teach Finch how to sign in
Egyptian! I could do weeks of laundry and plan meals for the next
millennium! I will be the Cat in the Hat of motherhood. I will be the
wife of the century! *Watch me balance a bottle of milk on my head. Watch me*
*stand on a ball. Watch me waffle and wiffle and chop, chop, chop, chop! Watch*
*me sandwich a manwich and play peekaboo. And that was not all I could do!*
*No, that was not all!*

Two weeks in, after taking the Ambien and the Benadryl booster
nightly like a good patient, my average sleep slips to four or five hours
a night. Some nights less. Hard to say. I'm a human skid mark, unsure
of where I start or end. In early May, after waking and swimming up
through the haze of medication, I realize it's my birthday: I'm turning
forty. The thought is like a wadded ball of paper thrown into a corner.
I see it through dull-lit eyes. Forty. What does that mean, forty? I'm

knocking solidly on the door of the aging—that's what it means. I'm not an adolescent anymore, not down the street buying a Coke at the corner store. I'm not riding the bus to school and wondering if my budding breasts are noticeable under my pale blue T-shirt. No, I'm on the front stoop of forty.

Sean and I decide that to commemorate this event, we will have a cake and sake party. We send out invitations. *Bring cake!* We enthuse. *Bring sake!* Sean will make salmon teriyaki and sticky rice because it's the only thing that sounds palatable to me. Everyone will get tipsy on Japanese rice wine, and the children, left to their own devices, will wander through the garden and torture small insects. We will all eat cake. We will toast to being forty and being alive.

We invite all our friends, including those we haven't seen since Finch was born. "Last chance for revelry," we tell people. "There's a second baby who's sixteen weeks along and already got one foot out the door!" I imagine us as carnival barkers corralling people into our sideshow: *See the exhausted and medicated forty-year-old! She's huge! She's a beach ball! And behind this curtain, the freaked-out husband! See him tuck, see him roll!*

Sean runs errands all morning. Salmon, check. Sake, check. Cake, check. He feels good with projects. They're predictable and conquerable. I put Finch in the Jonny Jump Up swing that Sean hung off the beam extending slightly off the back of the house. Finch jumps and jumps while I wind pieces of turquoise-colored diaphanous fabric around the base of the pear and apple trees in the backyard. I steal all the battery-powered candles from the front room and set them in a ring around each tree.

"It's the little things that make magic," I tell Finch, wafting one of the pieces of fabric in front of him. He stretches his hand out and his blue eyes go wild. It's a flying cobalt crane, a glittery gossamer float. I end up tying it just over his head so when a breeze comes he can watch it make little trails through the air.

My boyo is nearly a year old. He's been doing physical therapy for about nine months, and Jenny, his therapist, says he'll crawl any day. He's been doing this launch maneuver where he rocks unsteadily back and forth on all fours while trying to hurl himself forward. We're told this rock-and-hurl is a developmental stage. He's managed a few arm wiggles along with the rock-and-hurls, but—despite all our enthusiastic gesticulations and promises of Goldfish crackers—crawling is going nowhere fast.

Last week I asked Jenny if she thought we might have a chance of getting Finch walking by the time his sister arrives. The thought of having his hand in mine while he totters around gets me misty. My little boy, vertical, face looking up. My boy standing next to me, hand rummaging around in the Skittles and Hershey bars that are toddler height in the checkout line of the grocery store. *No, honey. No candy. We have pears, love. Pears!* And I'll pick him up and rub noses and he'll squirm free and run down the cereal aisle, bag of Skittles in hand with me loping after him, both of us giggling while shoppers turn to stare at the uncommon revelry, the unabashed joy. Oh, it will be beautiful.

Jenny smiles when I ask the question. She says that getting Finch walking in the next few months is a wonderful goal, really, but most kids with Down syndrome don't walk until they're at least two. Often longer. Finch has great gross motor skills and his legs aren't bowed, but he'll be rock-and-hurling for a while yet. *Right, then,* I think. *What's the hurry? Why am I in such a hurry to get this kid upright? Slow is good. Slow is a beautiful, teachable thing and I will learn to let it wash over me. Finch's rock-and-hurl will be genius! We'll weep with its very perfection. We'll YouTube it and there will be a collective sigh as the world is reminded of the glorious possibility of an unhurried life.*

After shopping for salmon and rice, balloons, and cups for sake, Sean lopes into the backyard. The garden looks like it was bombed by a group of renegade fairies. "Nice," he says, kissing me, one arm curling around my waist. "I'm going to make you the best birthday dinner you've ever had," he says into my neck. "And then I'm going to take your clothes off." He pulls back to look into my eyes and the heat's immediate. He does this to me. All he has to do is look at me with those eyes, whisper into my neck, and I'm lost.

"Take my clothes off," I say. "*Now.* Finch is napping." After playing with the streams of fabric I set up for him, Finch fell asleep, one cheek resting against the rope of the Jonny Jump Up, his arms limp. I tucked him into his crib and he curled around his teddy bear, fingers moving in slow circles around the tiny brown eyes.

Sean traces his finger across my collarbone, down the length of my already huge belly, to the elastic waistband of my pregnant jeans.

"Sexy," he says.

"Take my clothes off now," I say. I'm almost begging him. It's so seldom I'm not crushed by fatigue that when I feel good, my body's hungers slam me like a freight train. I try to press myself against him. This has the unfortunate effect of pushing him back against the counter as if I've hockey checked him. I try again, sliding my fingers the length of his zipper. "Come on," I say, getting on tiptoe to kiss him again. "I'll make it worth your while."

"Hold on there, Lolita. I'm making teriyaki for forty people." He grabs my hand and rubs my fingers over his lips. "We'll unwrap gifts later, okay?"

"Okay . . . yeah . . . okay." I feel stalled, adolescent heat crashing through my body. "Okay," I say, backing out of the kitchen. "You cook. Gifts later."

And when our friends come, it's magic. We haven't seen many of them for so long. "Hello, my God! Hello!" My dear friend Sedina, who dances in a local Samba group and does things on four-inch heels that take my breath away. Ivy arrives with a leather-bound book in which people can write birthday poems and wishes. I hug her hard, pour her a cup of sake, and give her the bottle. And then Jerome and Hollis arrive—the most energetic of my friends despite being late into their sixties—back after their trip to New Zealand, where they drove everywhere in an RV and woke one morning to watch a kea bird pull off the RV's windshield wipers and eat the rubber. "Hello, my God! The rubber? You're serious?" They're home for now, heading to India in the fall.

The yard begins filling up and the table overflows with custard tarts and cupcakes, *honjozo* and *namazake* and coarsely filtered *nigori* sakes. Children walk through the compost, swing around the pear trees, and steal bits of cake. Sean's sister and husband come with their kids. Jameson, six-year-old son to Sean's Frisbee friends, unwraps one of the apple trees and runs back and forth through the yard with a stream of fabric whipping in the wind behind him. Soon there's a line of kids chasing one after another, leaping over lavender bushes, throwing the fabric into the air to see who can catch it.

It's in this moment I realize how crushed I've been. Since taking Ambien, even on the worst nights, I've averaged enough sleep to keep me from losing my squash. My skin doesn't burn, and I can feel pleasure and colors and the sun. My God. I want this more than anything. Those months without sleep felt endless. Arms and legs jerking, memory loss, heart palpitations, and moods that shifted from blue to black in the space of a night. But tonight—God, tonight—I feel awe at my husband's heat, my boy, my friends. There's so much awe in being human. I want to bottle it and hold it close and never be dragged under the terror of sleepless waters again.

As the sun sinks toward the horizon, the garden glows gold. Sean brings out plate after plate of sticky rice and salmon. The smell is honey tang and fish, the smell of sex and spring. Everyone crowds around the tables, heaping spoonfuls onto their plates, grabbing more sake, laughing at the sudden crush of hungry bodies. I stand next to Sean, feeling his warmth. My fingers search for his hand and we stand together like this for a long time, fingers entwined, the soundtrack of the evening a joyful banter pulsing around us. Finally, Sean lets go and we move in different directions, weaving through the garden to find friends who slipped in after the crush. "Yes, Melissa's due at the end of October!

Ready? No, we're not ready but who's ever really ready? We're just jumping off the parental cliff again."

At the end of the evening, after the last round of sake is poured and downed and the last friend hugged, Sean and I stand looking into the garden.

"That was one fine party," Sean says. I nod. Candles flicker under the trees. Pieces of fabric lie strewn by the tomatoes and twined around tree branches. We move slowly, gathering plates and putting the empty sake bottles in the recycling. When the yard is cleared, we move into the house and then the bedroom. We lie together and I nestle my head against Sean's shoulder.

"Thank you," I say. "I think that's the best birthday I've ever had."

"I'm glad," he says, brushing a strand of hair from my face. And then he runs his lips across my forehead. His breath is slow and hot, and his mouth moves to the side of my neck and then over my belly and down and the heat rises again, fast and hard, and it fills the room.


DURING THE DAY my heart races. I'm taking the Ambien CR the nurse prescribed, but it's been nearly eight weeks and sleep has dropped down to four hours a night at best. You're not supposed to feel your heart race as if it's trying to find an exit, trying to find a way out of the birdcage of the ribs. One shouldn't feel these things. It's an indication that the wiring is off, something is jacked up, messages are being sent willy-nilly from the brain that have no bearing on what the body needs. I'll be standing at the window or rocking Finch in my arms and I'll drop suddenly, as if the cabin pressure has gone to nothing. I'm a fainting woman. I'm a drifting woman without a chaise lounge, so I stand near the couch, the chair, the bed, one hand always at the ready to catch myself. I don't know if this is the medication or the pregnancy. I want to sleep. This is all I know.

At night, consciousness pushes through like mud in a sieve. Some-time after my first prescription, I burst through the pharmaceutical haze and wandered around the house half-cocked. I sat on the couch watching the little clock on the side table move from twelve o'clock to one o'clock to two. At 2:30 a.m. I freaked out. The insomnia was the hungry caterpillar, the insatiable larva in one of the books I'd been reading to Finch. I needed to call someone. No. There was no one to call. Who would one call at 2:30 in the morning to discuss such things? I decided it would be best if I just got into the car and drove. This was a brilliant idea. The car would be safe. I wouldn't bother anyone, and I could drive to Utah's south desert with all the pretty sandstone arches. Maybe I'd hike. Maybe I'd get lost like the famed Everett Ruess, the young artist who set out into the Utah desert in 1934 and was never seen again. That sounded lovely—me dissolving into the desert like Ruess, becoming a forty-year-old mystery. Maybe I'd buy a donut.

I grabbed my keys and was just opening the front door to leave when Sean stopped me. You can hear everything in our little house, so I try to creep around like a mouse to avoid waking Sean or Finch. I don't remember Sean stumbling from the bedroom to find me, hand on the door. I don't remember a tussle or getting back into bed. I don't remember if Sean was angry because he had to get up in the morning and load his landscaping truck with dogwood trees. Perhaps he just led me gently by the elbow, nudging me like an orderly with an elderly patient who'd been found wandering the hall in their skivvies. Regardless, I returned to bed and lay down, consciousness fading to black. Later, I dreamed of a road, desolate and distant, stretching to an impossible horizon.

I don't remember us talking about it in the morning. It seems like a thing a couple would talk about, but my memory is turning to vapor. And Sean doesn't like to talk about things that are in any way uncertain. I try to keep conversations to the empirical—the orange peels on the table, the diapers that need to be restocked, the coffee grounds, the plants that are dying to be watered. Soon even this begins to dry up.

# BLUR

*July 2009*

AT MONTH SIX OF MY PREGNANCY, Finch turns a year old and moves out of the realm of the rock-and-hurl into full crawling. He's no speed demon but the boy is solid. The first day he makes it from the red rug in the front room to the hallway that leads first to our tucked bedroom and then the kitchen. The next day he makes it from the red rug all the way through the hallway, and into the kitchen—a ten-foot improvement, for which I believe he should get some kind of award. The first time he stayed up after his rock-and-hurl, he looked at me with a surprised expression as if to say, *Holy shit—did you know this was actually going to work?*

I start crawling with him for little bits of time during the day. My belly seems to be contracting all the time, and being on all fours helps. Being anything other than upright helps. The day Finch makes it to the kitchen on his own, it's as if he's never seen a floor before. He stops and stares like it's the Grand Canyon. I'm hefting plates into the high cabinet when I hear the sound. I turn and realize Finch has discovered the cat's dish of tiny crunchy stars. He's facedown in the bowl, ecstatic.

Later that afternoon, Ivy stops by with a birthday present for Finch: a tiny red shirt that has a print of Alfred Hitchcock with a raven sitting on his shoulder. For years, I dreamed of being a cinematographer like Hitchcock's Leslie Robert Burks. I loved the precise measure of scenes to create tension and the innovative use of light. I envisioned Burks as a visual philosopher. He inquired as to the precise emotion a scene was meant to convey and sculpted the light on the set to reveal it. He was measured, methodical, and unwaveringly mathematical in his arrangements. Each scene was a formula and each formula led to an inescapable truth.

I make Ivy mint tea and we sit at the kitchen table while Finch sleeps. It's been four months since the *Wasatch Journal* folded, and in that time not only has Ivy not found a job but her husband, Jack, was let go from his work as an administrator at a local high school. We've all fallen into the recession abyss and Jack and Ivy are scrabbling hard, trying to find work in the slippery talus field of our once shiny and bubbled America. And despite being scared, Ivy remains hopeful. She's an academic. She received a PhD in history from Brown. Under normal circumstances, employers would be hot in the pants to hire her. But neither she nor Jack has found anything. Four months in, they've received one and only one offer. Ivy sits with her hands wrapped around her tea and tells me that this summer she's going to be a kitchen bitch in Alaska. They're going to fly north to work at a private corporate resort outside Anchorage.

"It'll be an adventure," she says.

I nod and refill her tea. All my thoughts in the past months of trying to get work in the magazine industry have evaporated. My life has become day and night and keeping Finch alive. I'm not an artist mother. I don't sparkle over the pot roast or rock the mama blog. I'm a couch sitter, a fly banging against a window, a watcher of clocks. I don't know how I'll ever find my way out of this. And Ivy's determined cheer only amplifies the anguish I push away like something rotting. I tell none of this to Ivy. I don't want to add my weight to hers. "Adventure," I say. "It'll be amazing."

One week after the public schools let out, Jack and Ivy leave for Alaska.


I FEEL MORE and more closed in, as if the very walls of the house are shrinking. I've gone from averaging seven hours of sleep a night to five to three. By September, four months after my first prescription, I'm again averaging two and a half hours. *Two and a half.* It's inhuman. Even with the pharmaceutical giants and their golden pills, on some nights I don't sleep at all and merely walk from room to hazy room in a cloud of doped-up anxiety.

With only two months until the baby is due, Sean decides he wants a night out with his friends. He just wants to sit and drink beer on tap and not think about things. "Go," I say. "Have a wonderful time." Beer and man talk and laughter will be great medicine. "Go." An hour after he leaves, anxiety creeps in. Sean is not a soothing presence in the house, but he's a tall, athletic man, and I feel so very weak. Despite his constant dark moods, his withdrawal from me, and his frustrations with my insomnia, at least he's got weight. He'd protect me and the son he adores if someone crept into the house.

And the truth is, I've had fears of break-ins since I was a child. I remember being ten years old and lying in bed, charting my routes of escape. I wondered what I would do if someone tried to hurt my mother or brother. Would I fight? Would I slide through the window near my bed and run through the black night for help? When Sean leaves, my old fears resurface. I tell myself I'm being irrational, but the night rises, dark and alien. Finch falls asleep in the crib we bought and set up in the basement. The video monitor shows his little body crawling around in sleep. I sit on the couch in the living room near the front door, waiting. And then it's ten. And then eleven. I pick up the book in front of me, attempting normalcy. The words blur in front of my eyes. Eleven thirty. I rub my fingers over the couch's tan microfiber. Midnight.

I look toward the big window. I look at the door next to it that leads right out to the street. The back door has a wide hole cut into the bottom of it that the previous owner installed. There's nothing but a vinyl flap over the hole for a dog we do not have. This house is permeable, flimsy. If someone wanted to break in, someone who was watching the house and waiting, a can opener would be the most they'd require. Maybe a pocketknife. And really, if they opened the gate leading to the backyard, they'd only need to shimmy through the dog door and there I'd be, in the kitchen or by the stair. I'd blink. I'd think about knives and protecting my son, but I'd be unable to move. I might hurl my huge and pregnant body at them, hoping for a block, a lucky strike if they were unsuspecting. But no, there's no way I'd escape. I'd most likely freeze like a deer in front of an approaching car. I'd stand shivering, easy prey for some crackhead who'd crawled in looking for cash. I'd see his eyes and know I was done for. I'd want to scream, but fear would be like cotton in my throat.

I freeze. My heart slams in my chest, trying to get out, trying to get anywhere but here. Sean will be home soon. I know it. There is no crackhead shimmying through the dogless dog door. No one is busting the lock on the front door. I'm suffering the paranoia of the pregnant. It's just Finch and me in a quiet house on a quiet street. I move from the couch to the bedroom and look at the video monitor. Finch hasn't moved. The blanket curls around his small body. No one has stolen him and sold him to an underground ring of thugs who will do unmentionable things. I breathe in front of the monitor. The air has grown thin. When did it get so thin, this air? I pace and sit. The monitor flickers ominously.

And then I hear it: a small sound in the kitchen, something scraping across the floor. My body floods with adrenaline. *Jesus Christ, someone is in the house.* They've been watching, and they know Sean has gone for beers. They'll hurt Finch and I won't be able to stop them. There will be blood on the walls. Holy shit, I can't breathe. Another small scrape. I can't *breathe*. Someone's *here*.

Our black cat, Goose, saunters into the bedroom and jumps on the bed. I startle and bump my elbow on the bed frame. Goose's little tongue licks the crunchy stars we feed him from the corners of his mouth. This would normally be hilarious, this realization that Goose was the intruder and the scraping sound I'd heard merely his cat bowl moving against the floor. I imagine telling Sean. I imagine us laughing. But I feel like I'm going to throw up and the air is still so thin.

I pace a slow track from the bedroom to the front door and then back again through the house to the kitchen and the stairs leading down to Finch's crib. This house is so small. There's a butcher knife in the kitchen. I grab the knife and begin repeatedly walking the length of the house, from front door to back, counting my breaths, talking myself off the edge of the cliff. I've been a rock climber and a sensitive poet but never someone so riddled with anxiety I fall to pieces the minute my husband leaves. I don't recognize this woman, fragile as spun glass.

*It's the Ambien*, I think, the idea rising out of the depths. *It's the Ambien. How many months have I been on it? Four? Five? Is that okay? Did the nurses say anything about long-term use? No.* I begin to argue with myself. *No, it's me. I'm beyond exhausted and I have a baby downstairs and this street is not the safest. There were two break-ins last month. That apartment building on the corner is a haven for dealers. It hasn't been a huge problem, but still . . .*

Humiliation washes over me. I put the knife down and keep walking. *Breathe in for four, out for six. Build a mantra. Hum the song of yourself. Do something.*

*You used to do yoga daily*, I remind myself. *You've traveled to third world countries alone. You've fought off bandits in Central America and gone rock climbing in Thailand. You've chased away monkeys from your tent by candlelight. You've run fifty miles and more without stopping. You've run for your life.*

Near the back door, a cluster of contractions doubles me over. I tuck into a ball, my hands flat against the floor. The doctors don't know why I'm having so many contractions. They don't know why I'm having heart palpitations or insomnia their drugs can't crush for more than a few weeks at a time. They don't know a fucking thing. Tears puddle on the floor. I crouch like this for an eternity. Then the door creaks open.

I startle at footsteps down the hall. My body half turns and I lock eyes with Sean. I see what he sees: his wife crouched in a ball near the back door, eyes wet and wide with panic.

"What the hell's going on?"

"Please don't go out again," I say, my voice constricted, light as air. "Please . . . I was so scared, and the contractions aren't stopping, and I'm just . . ."

"I was out for *beers*," Sean says, irritated, as though my actions are incomprehensible to him. He searches my face. "What—did you think I wasn't going to come home?"

"No, no. I just . . . everything hurts so much, and I feel so vulnerable." I start crying again. "I'm sorry, I know you just wanted a night out and I so wanted you to have a night out, but . . ." I burn with humiliation. He's angry and confused. I want to give him a normal life and I'm giving him a wife who clings to him with a postapocalyptic desperation.

Sean stands and stares, his body rigid. His face is a frozen swirl of emotion—beers, friends, and then this? Where's the woman he married? Who is this fragile and broken creature? He hesitates and then walks toward me.

Shame consumes my face. "I was scared."

"Okay," he says. "It's okay. Let's just go to sleep."

I lie in bed next to him, cursing. This will all be over once the baby's born. Until then, I promise myself I won't be such a freak. It's pregnancy. Pregnancy's hard. Whatever. I fold into a wash of self-condemnation. I lie awake.

# REDEMPTION AND
# THE MANGA CHICK

*September–October 2009*

TWO DAYS AFTER MY NIGHT OF panic, an idea hits. It's a brilliant plan that will offer joy and hope and redemption from the guilt that consumes me. I'm so happy with this plan, I immediately get Dirk, Sean's best friend from high school who now lives in Seattle, in on it. The two grew up together near Sun Valley, Idaho, and have remained in touch since then. I put Finch on the floor and construct a circle around him with stuffed puppies, bears, and unicorns. He'll have to crawl over them to get out. Finch lies next to the unicorn and fingers its glittery purple face. I call Dirk.

"Dirk, hey—it's Melissa."

"Melissa, sweetheart! Hold just a sec. Alex, don't hit your sister." He pauses. I hear walking and then the wail of his youngest daughter. I wait. Dirk is the tallest, blondest man I've ever met. He has three daughters—eight, six, and two—who are equally tall and blond. They are a house of beautiful, Amazonian creatures. Even the two-year-old seems to have sprung from the womb looking like a kindergartner.

"Sorry about that," Dirk says when he's back on the phone. "Alex thinks it's funny to hide Willow's pacifier on the trampoline outside. Willow was trying to get out the front door."

"Awww, poor Willow," I say. "It's so sad when they move out of the potted plant stage." Dirk guffaws. The sound of his laugh could carry miles. Dirk is the guy you always want at a party. He'll convince everyone to do shooters and then bust into the neighbor's pool to swim naked. When I tell him I want to put together a boy's trip to Seattle for Sean's upcoming fortieth birthday, he's euphoric. He needs a trip, too, he says. This is beyond perfect. It's genius.

"We should try to get this together for the first weekend in October," I tell him. "The girl's due October twenty-eighth. I can bring my mom in and we can send Sean off with a plane ticket and nothing else."

"Damn," Dirk says. "You know, I'm pretty sure I can get tickets to the Seattle Mariners. I know a guy who can set us up behind home plate." His voice has motion. I've pitched the ball and he's hit it out of the park. "Let me get on the horn. This can be a reunion tour. My God"—he's nearly out of breath—"I can look at houses on Lopez Island. Fuck! Lopez Island! We can get the boys together before we turn geriatric."

"Get on the horn," I say. We're both brimming with excitement. "We don't have much time."

We hang up agreeing to communicate via email so we can stay in hourly contact. Finch has made it over the unicorn and his little diapered body is heading for the cat dish. I pick him up and hold him suspended in front of me. Those eyes. "I love you, Finch," I say, still holding him. He looks down at his feet and then up at me, smiling. I tuck my hand under his bottom and sit at the kitchen table with the computer. I have several hours until Sean gets back from work. Fall cleanup often puts Sean in a bad mood. He spends days raking and bagging rotting leaves and he just wants to be done with it all. I put Finch on my lap and give him the unicorn.

"Look, Finch," I say as I look up vacation rentals. "Water! Trees!" I point to the images on the screen. "We're going to surprise him, aren't we, sweetie? Daddy has no idea what's coming." In minutes, I find a huge house overlooking the Strait of Juan de Fuca. Six large bedrooms. Hot tub. Private beach. Moss so thick you could hide in it. Vistas of ocean water and a tangerine sky.

I email the information to Dirk. Two hours later I receive an email back that three friends from high school are on board. With Dirk's powers of persuasion and the need of forty-year-old men to drink deep from the kegger of nostalgia, it looks as if we just may pull this together.

In five hours, Dirk emails me that ten guys are on board. He's making reservations for the first weekend in October. We're out-of-our-minds giddy, so excited to give something big to Sean—a vacation from all of this. *Just hang on*, I think. *Please, just hang on until the end of October so I can give this to Sean.* I purchase a Seattle Mariners baseball cap from eBay. They're playing the Texas Rangers on October 2. It's a go.

THE SEATTLE MARINERS cap just arrived. There's a knock at the door, and when I open it, there's a marvelous light rain. I grab the box and look up. Thunder rolls through the dark sky and wind pushes its hands through the trees. Inside, I take the hat out and put it on Finch's head. We snuggle on the couch and watch the rain as he tips his head back and forth to feel the fabulous polyester cap slide. I pull the cap up, playing peekaboo, and he leans his head back to look at me. Eyes like the cosmos—white, then blue and more blue, a giant rim of blue. He sits back, shucks off the hat, and grabs his feet, which look like miniature apricots.

I drink in days like these—days when I don't feel frayed and adrenaline soaked. Despite the Ambien and the recommended booster of Benadryl, sleep now feels like a game of chance, a roll of the dice. Snake eyes and I'm in luck. A one and a two, no dice and I wander the dimly lit hall. This is my temporary fate, I think. Soon I'll give birth to my baby girl and I won't feel knifed and I'll never take a pill again. Whatever hormonal wreckage has occurred with this pregnancy will calm. The waters will still. I'll have my baby and my body and I'll once again be someone who doesn't panic when night comes.

After lunch of yam and little bits of cheese and peaches, I put Finch in his crib for a nap. Upstairs, I put the Mariners cap in a shoebox and shove it under the bed. I kick a couple of shirts in front of the box for effect. Sean will never even look. And even if he does find the cap, he won't be tipped off. He isn't a fan of the Seattle Mariners. Not many people are unless you live in Seattle and get whipped into a froth over bad baseball. Last year the Mariners were dead last in the American League West.

ON THE DAY before his departure, Sean comes home exhausted. He's spent the day raking and hefting leaves, pruning rosebushes, and mowing lawns that have surged past their proper one-and-a-half-inch height. I tell him to take his shoes off, to rest for a while. I've cooked his favorite: coconut curry chicken with jasmine rice.

I know I'll have to work hard to convince Sean to go. This is part of the delight. Sean will look at my belly, knowing that at thirty-six weeks our girl could come at any time. He'll look at me with apprehension, but I won't accept no for an answer. I'll be strong. He'll see my determination and his heart will go tender with overwhelm. Love will be the salve to our exhausted bodies. I'll be a woman of virtue and strength, and our happiness will smoke between us. I hum around the kitchen with an energy I haven't felt in months. I let the rice breathe, add the curry paste to heavy coconut milk, keep Finch busy with the great riot of stuffed animals and blocks.

I realize in some shadowed portion of my mind that I'm propelled by guilt. My neediness repels me. Feeling weak and dependent is a torture neither Sean nor I can stand. At night I'm plagued with a persistent condemnation that even as a stay-at-home-mama cliché, I can't keep up. Giving this trip, when I'm as weak as I've ever been, is my way to feel strong again.

I've promised to email Dirk a report this evening once I give Sean his gift. Sean's scheduled to leave for Seattle tomorrow morning at 10:00 a.m. My mom will get in at half past noon. By the time Finch has his second nap, Sean will be in a bar downtown with five additional friends. By dinnertime they'll be behind home plate at the Mariners game. Ten more friends will arrive at the game, each holding a beer or a hot dog. They'll act stunned, but by that time the jig will be up. The next morning they'll all leave for Lopez Island.

SEAN SLUMPS ON the couch as I stir the chicken curry. After a few minutes he goes out to the shed. It's October and not quite freezing but close. He's probably smoking pot. I don't care that he smokes, but I've been noticing it makes him vague and far away. I'm changing Finch on the bed when Sean comes in. The refrigerator door opens.

"The beer's for dinner!" I yell.

"Dinner's ready, isn't it?" Sean yells back, opening the beer.

I bring Finch into the kitchen and put him in his high chair.

"We're having coconut curry chicken," I say, raising my eyebrows.

"Nice," Sean says, nuzzling Finch, who's grabbed at Sean's light beard to run his little hands over the man stubble.

We eat with me feeding Finch bits of mango from my plate and Sean silently sipping his beer, eyes pinned to the window leading to the backyard. When we're done, I pick up our plates and deposit them in the sink. I turn and face him, holding the thin metal border on the counter behind me.

"What?" he asks.

"I've got an early birthday present for you."

"Oh, yeah?"

"Yeah." I smile and go into the bedroom. I place the shoebox in front of Sean. Finch stares.

"Should I open it now?" Sean asks.

"*Yes*, you should open it now," I say. I roll my eyes for effect and nudge his leg.

Sean opens the box. "Seattle Mariners," he says. "Um . . . thanks?" He puts the hat on Finch's head.

He has no idea. I feel ecstatic, outside myself with excitement. A boy's weekend trip on a beautiful island is the last thing he'd imagine I'd give him for his birthday—especially with me so close to delivering our girl. I feel triumphant.

"I have one more surprise," I say, grabbing the envelope I've hidden on top of the fridge. I place it neatly in front of him and sit down.

"What's this?" he asks.

"Open it."

Sean opens the envelope and pulls out the plane tickets. After a full ten seconds of bewildered staring he gives a tremendous whoop.

"Seattle?" he yells, incredulous, his eyes wide with disbelief. "Oh my fucking God, Seattle? Tomorrow? Are you kidding me?" Then he jumps up and runs into the bedroom to start packing.


"It's my fault," I say to my mom. I haven't seen her since Christmas, and while we've talked on the phone about my drag of insomnia, I don't think she truly understands. I know she tries, but her difficulty in making ends meet in California engulfs her in a dark cloud. Our talks are often short and awkward, with both of us wanting to connect but forever missing. We're sitting in the living room, watching snow dump out of a dark sky as I battle a cocktail of self-congratulation and self-loathing.

"I'm an idiot. I mean, who gives a gift they want someone to refuse? Who does that? I'm so fucked-up. I'm so tragically fucked-up right now."

"Oh, honey." My mom puts her hand on my leg.

"I should be happy," I continue. "I mean, I *am*. Happy. I just wish he hadn't been so out-of-his-mind euphoric. He was packed within ten minutes, Mom. Maybe less. There was no hesitation, no 'Are you going to be okay, babe?' I don't think he even asked me a question after that beyond wondering what time we had to leave for the airport."

"Sweetie, you gave an incredible gift. I'm sure he only went because he knew I'd take care of you." She pauses. I stare at the fury of flakes outside the window. Finch sits on my lap, staring at his hands as if sea anemones have suddenly sprouted from the ends of his wrists.

"Hey, why don't we plan on having a yummy dinner tomorrow night? It's too dark in this house. I'll take care of my grandson and you can just relax."

"Did I tell you he was euphoric?"

"Yes, you did."

"God, I'm lame. I am so, so lame."

"You're not lame, honey. You're exhausted, and this pregnancy has taken a lot out of you. I'm going to go make reservations for tomorrow night. You rest and tomorrow we'll go somewhere nice. This carpet is filthy."

The next day stretches like a long, tight string. Nothing to do but watch the snow and try to extinguish the feeling that I am, without a doubt, a complete fuck-up as a wife and a human.

Mom takes Finch and me to dinner at Sprouts, a vegan diner in the south end of the city with retro vinyl booths and waiters sheathed in tattoos. None of us is vegan, but Mom is always trying new diets to combat her tendency to eat entire cakes when depression hits. We eat Happy Teriyaki bowls with spongy squares of vegetable protein. The squares are supposed to give the impression of meat but are so far from meat, so very protozoan in their appearance, they look like a chicken fried steak someone would buy in the early-morning hours at a Denny's restaurant.

Mom jokes that she's been addicted to everything and given up everything in her lifetime: cocaine, alcohol, Diet Coke, in that order. She went into rehab when I was a senior in high school. It was the late 1980s and there weren't that many rehab centers back then.

Later that night, after Finch falls asleep, she recounts the story of what pushed her into rehab. She'd admitted herself in October 1986, so every year since then we revisit it. It's become a kind of ritual for her, for us—something to help her remember where she was and how far she's come. Every November we celebrate the date she was released as a birthday.

"I'll never forget seeing you walk to Matt's house," she says. I'd moved into my boyfriend's parents' garage to escape her cocaine-fueled rages. "I was standing in that liquor store, buying my gallon of Scotch, and you just walked by with your shaved head and those thrift store clothes." She pauses. "I never want to feel that way again."

She talks about how, after buying the Scotch, she'd spent the night drinking until the bottle emptied. She held the pawnshop pistol she'd bought weeks earlier in her hands, contemplating suicide. In the early-morning hours she drove to an isolated beach near Half Moon Bay, a quaint coastal town thirty miles south of San Francisco. She'd tucked the pistol in her pants and walked the sand until her feet touched water. She was going to do it right there—pull the trigger and leave her body to the salt and fish. The pain was unbearable. For years she described her sudden urge to throw the gun into the ocean as a gift from angels. Now she says she knew she couldn't leave us. She'd left us alone with her alcoholism and drug use; she couldn't add suicide.

After throwing the gun as hard as she could, she drove herself to a bleak hospital in San Mateo, California. She had a thirty-day inpatient stint and came out like spun glass. Back then, her addiction was an abstraction to me. It took decades for me to understand how profoundly the drugs had fueled her rages and isolation. All I knew was I felt both scared of her and desperate for her love. I was an addict's daughter—constantly on eggshells and filled with my own dynamite.

And in the darkest places in me I condemned her. I saw her as weak, never fully understanding what it took to be a single mother of two—a single mother battling unacknowledged depression. She came out of rehab in debt, filled with shame, and jobless. But she never relapsed. Other addictions floated around, landing on shopping binges when she was making money and dollar store bags of M&M's when she wasn't, but she never drank again.

As our conversation winds down, I promise Mom I will sleep. I stare at the walls. My voicemail's empty. No messages of concern, no tidbits of love or thanks. I feel crushed at my own smallness, at how much I want my husband to be grateful and worried. I want him to check on me daily and shower me with adoration. And because he doesn't, because he packed for the trip with the intensity of a military man out on furlough, I feel bereft and naked under a hot blanket of shame. All I can do is hold the small part inside of me and not hate it, not condemn it for showing up, for reminding me it's part of who I am.

I don't think I can stand much more. That night the contractions are so strong, my hips sear, which the nurse-midwives tell me is normal. But a new body oddity has cropped up. I can't get away from the smell of ashtrays. It follows me everywhere—to the bathroom, to the kitchen, outside. I call the midwives, but they have no answer. *Ashtrays, huh?* They give me the medical shrug. *Pregnancy does all kinds of funky things to the body. It'll probably go away.*

Saturday afternoon, Sean calls. He and the guys are waiting for the ferry. He tells me about running into Slide and Johnny on the plane to Seattle and how convincing they were, walking away after collecting their bags and telling Sean to text later that night if he could meet for a drink. After Dirk picked him up, they had lunch at a burger joint and then Dirk said that they should stop by this cool bar before going back to Dirk's place. When they got there, Johnny and Slide were in a booth doing shooters with three of Sean's friends from high school.

"At that point," Sean says, "I knew something was up, but no one would tell me where we were going. Eight guys showed up at the Mariners game, maybe ten. They were in a row of seats behind home plate eating hot dogs before we even got there. Fuck, it was awesome. They even got me a bat."

"A bat?"

"Yeah. Dirk got one of those old-school wooden bats and all the guys signed it at the bar afterwards."

"Really?" I breathe in with one of the contractions. "That's great, sweetie." Mom has ventured out in the snow with Finch to buy some milk and cake. I breathe out.

"Phil actually met some hyper-sexed manga chick at the bar. You remember Phil? He was at the wedding. Anyway, the guys didn't even tell me about Lopez Island until this morning."

"I know. It's going to be great. Happy birthday, honey."

"Thanks. Fuck, the ferry leaves in ten minutes and Phil's still MIA. He's probably at the manga chick's house. I swear that guy has no shame."

"Maybe it's love," I say, trying for a joke.

"Yeah," Sean laughs, "with him, it's always love . . . Listen," he says, his voice tensing, "I need to be fully transparent with you about something."

"Oh," I say, my whole body on high alert. He needs to be transparent. "What is it?"

He begins a rambling confession. "I partied way too much last night," he says. "It was stupid, I know . . . but I was with the guys and everyone was into it and it was just so easy."

"Oh?" I'm so hypersensitive from sleep deprivation, I steel myself. I have no idea what he's about to say, and I tell myself not to overreact. Then again, I've been so exhausted for so long, I don't know what a normal reaction is to *anything*. I'm lost in the struggle to just try to make it through each day.

"Yeah. I partied way too much," Sean says. He doesn't sound apologetic. He sounds guilty. It feels as if he's run into a confessional booth for a quick fix, wants to empty his pockets of shame onto the floor and get back to the fun. "It was just . . . well . . . I just wanted you to know . . . I think it's important that we're transparent with each other."

"Oh," I say again, and we pause. I assume he's launched into full disclosure because he wants me to absolve him of his immense partying or he hopes I'll give him some Hail Marys before he heads out. It's like pond scum has just sluiced into my lap. I'm holding my hands aloft, trying not to touch it.

"So anyway," he repeats, "I just want us to . . . you know . . . be transparent."

I stumble over a half-hearted okay but I wish he hadn't said anything. If he'd tried to get the manga chick to touch his penis or to drink beer out of his mouth, then yes, transparency would be important. But this transparency isn't about me—it's about him. He makes his statement of wanting to be transparent and waits. He does not ask me if I've slept. He does not apologize or express any kind of regret. He asks no questions regarding how I feel about what he's told me. He states his facts and I can take them or leave them. And then the ferry arrives and he has to get off the phone in a hurry, which is just as well. I feel gross.

When Mom gets back, I tell her Sean called but I don't say anything about his confession. I stay on the couch, slumped and sodden and eating the small bits of cake she offers. She keeps giving me worried glances while trying to help Finch stack blocks, but he just wants to swipe the towers with his hand. I know how he feels. I want to break everything I can get my hands on, but I can't even stand up. I have nothing left. I sit on the couch, managing contractions and swiping at the rivulets of tears running down my face.

MOM AND I are making eggs when the phone rings. I grab it, ridiculous in my hope that it might be Sean. I haven't heard from Sean, and don't expect to hear from him while he's on the island, but I so want to hear that he misses me or is worried or that he wants to know how I feel about the partying. Something. But it's not Sean; it's Hollis. She and Jerome are back from their trip to India. Her voice rings out warm and radiant. It's a warmth I haven't felt for so long, I can feel my whole body lean in.

I've known this couple for over a decade. I was an eager young reporter when I walked into the University of Utah's theater department to do an article on their avant-garde rendition of Euripides. Hollis was the head of marketing and we talked for so long, I completely forgot to interview the play's director. I had to call back the next day to cover my tracks and we giggled like young girlfriends on a playground, though she and Jerome are my mom's age. We've been friends ever since, and I now consider Hollis, Jerome, and their three adult children my adopted family.

She tells me that, while in India, she and Jerome attended the wedding of one of the innumerable exchange students they've hosted over the years. Incredible, she says. Murali and his betrothed's names were written in fire in the square. The whole thing was lit like Vegas but with incense and fireworks going off and everyone dancing in the street for miles and miles. And then there was a banquet that lasted until four in the morning. Imagine! After that, they went to Vrindavan, the sacred city of widows, where over fifteen thousand women who'd lost their husbands live, and gave devotion to Lord Krishna. Such beauty, she says. All of India is filled with it. They want to tell me everything and they have hundreds of photos. She insists that Mom and I come for a late brunch. They have gifts and they have croissants. They can't wait to see me and hear how the baby is doing. "Please come."

And so we do. Mom and I heft Finch into the car and when we arrive at their front door the social contagion is immediate. Hollis hugs me with her whole body and I lean in, remembering that after twenty seconds of this kind of hugging the brain begins secreting happy chemicals, the limbic system jumping for joy, like a gleeful child on a king-size bed. It's in this house, I realize, I've experienced undiluted love.

This house, which is filled with photos and art from all over the world, every corner a reverie of sorts, is saturated with the love of art, travel, and family. An antique printer's tray hangs vertically on a wall and is stuffed with small photos, matchbooks, and collages. Over the doorway to the sitting room is an Australian wood carving bought at a small shop decades ago. A delicate antique table sitting at the entrance to the backyard overflows with orchids, succulents, and a sleeping stone head. Years ago Hollis decorated the chandelier above the dining room table with shards of glass—cobalt, cinnamon, azure, rose—all collected from the glassblower Dale Chihuly's driveway and hung dangling from delicate golden threads. This is the kind of beauty that transforms because it's birthed from love. Beauty emanates from every corner like a warm breeze, so tangible, it's a presence.

I haven't thought of the philosophers or much of anything lately, but I can almost feel the nineteenth-century German philosopher Hegel standing next to me, reveling. *You're right, Hegel*, I think, closing my eyes for a moment. *You understand the yearning of the heart. The point of art isn't a grasping at imitation. It's to show us what divine human freedom looks like.* I open my eyes, taking in the pulse of beauty around me. *And it looks like this.*

I walk to the kitchen, putting Finch down to let him show off his crawling. Jerome tells Finch he'll be an Olympian and then walks over to place the gentlest of kisses on my lips. From anyone else this would feel too intimate, but from Jerome, who is like a father to me, it's like the most tender of hugs. "Welcome," he says, smiling. This man, who is a psychiatrist—someone who deals with emotional instability and psychosis every day and who could by extension be himself unstable or bitter or worse—is deeply compassionate in his understanding of the human condition. He looks into my eyes and says *Welcome* and his kindness fills my very cells. Hollis and Jerome welcome my mother, giving her long hugs in turn and telling her how wonderful it is to see her. Mom has met them once before, but it's been years. *Welcome, welcome!*

I grab Finch and we gather at the large island near the stove, watching Hollis make curried eggs and laughing as Finch grabs at Hollis's hair.

The warmth of the house plumps me, making me stouter and stronger. Mom asks Jerome about India. She's never been there, never traveled much, actually, but someday perhaps she, too, will go, she says.

At the table, after the croissants and eggs have been eaten, after the stories of India have been told with gusto, the pictures of widows and the betrothed shown, Hollis asks me to come up to the bedroom. She's bought a sari, she says, the typical dress for women of India. She must show me. I give Finch to Mom and follow Hollis upstairs. She sits on the bed and pats the spot next to her.

"How are you doing?" she asks, her voice suddenly serious. "Jerome and I have been worried."

"Oh, Hollis," I say, sitting next to her. I don't know how to tell her how absolutely crushed I am, how terrified I am for my daughter, how every day I worry that I won't make it. "Hollis . . . I . . ."

"You can tell me," she says, her bright blue eyes full of worry. "It looks like the baby has dropped. Are you sleeping?"

"Yes. A little. I mean, I was for a while. But now . . . no, not really."

Hollis sighs and squeezes my leg. "We just don't know what to *do*. I can't imagine what this has been like. Tell me, is there anything? What can we do?"

I stare at the floor. "I don't think there's anything anyone can do. The doctors don't know. I just have to hang in there. I think if I can make it a few more weeks . . ." I stroke the fabric on the bedspread. Subtle gold threads lace through some kind of flower—petunias? No, these flowers are big and succulent. Poppies?

"I've been thinking," Hollis says, her hand now resting on my thigh. I touch her index finger with mine. Her fingers are so delicate, long and tapered.

"Oh?"

"I used to be a labor coach," she says. "Back in Baltimore. Did you know that?"

"I didn't . . . no, I don't think you've told me that."

"I trained for quite a while."

"Really?"

"I want you to consider having me as your labor coach," she says. "I think I could help."

I stroke Hollis's soft fingers. Peonies, I think. The bedspread is like a garden of peonies. I feel my body relax into the warmth. Such incredible beauty.

"I'll make little ice chips of tea and juice. And you can call me anytime. You know what a night owl I am. I mean it—anytime. I'm here for you."

"Oh, Hollis," I say. "Yes, yes, I'd love that. Thank you." I can feel the gathering storm of bees under my skin. I'm so tired. And in this moment, gratitude is the balm keeping me together. I'll make it. Beauty is in this house and I'm breathing it like oxygen. I hold Hollis's tapered fingers.

"Thank you," I say, my eyes surrendering to a flow of tears. I'm stunned in the presence of her deep generosity. It's as if another room in a house has opened that I had no idea existed. I'm awkward at the threshold, stunned there are people who love this way—stunned they've invited me in.

# POOL OF THE PELVIS

*October 2009*

1:24 A.M.

My water breaks like a popgun and I know. Finally. Our girl's coming. She's ready for her exit. I nudge Sean and he mumbles in his sleep, turning away from me. I get up for a towel and spread it on the bed. *I'll sit on the couch*, I think. My life has been this couch, watching the play of weather outside, the bookcase in the corner, the sage-colored walls. I can wait a bit longer.

I try meditating, but I'm too excited. Nothing could be as bad as this pregnancy has been, and now it is over. I'll push my girl out, Hollis will hold my hand, and Sean and I will weep with relief that our girl is here and the insomnia will be gone.

I feel a familiar rise in intensity that signifies I'm in active labor. At 3:00 a.m. I begin timing the contractions. Still four minutes apart. It's been like this off and on for months. I remember the nurse who monitored my fetal stress tests telling me that it would suck for me, but my girl was fine. I tell myself that if I've endured contractions this long, I can take it for another day or so. I make some tea with honey. I sit. Just under four. At 5:00 a.m., I walk into the bedroom. A knife draws its blade across my belly.

"Sean?" Muffled rustling as his body moves under the covers. I take a deep breath. "*Sean*."

It's the statement that wakes him. Clear and strong.

"Huh?"

"My water broke."

"Oh, shit," he says, blinking. "When?"

"Three and a half hours ago."

"Okay." He shakes his head, driving away sleep. "Do we need to go to the hospital?"

"Not yet. Just get ready, okay?" I grip the dresser. A contraction pulses, hot and fierce. My uterus should be like a pump: squeeze and release, squeeze and release. But something's off. Something won't let go.

"Yeah," he says, fumbling with the comforter. "Okay. I'm up." He swings his long legs over the side of the bed and sits, staring at the wall. After a minute he stands and pulls on some pants. "You okay?"

"Just a contraction," I say. "I'm going to go sit on the couch."

Sean makes a cup of coffee and puts my bag by the front door. He calls Christina, who's been waiting for this call for weeks. She'll stay at the house with Finch while we're at the hospital. Sean comes to sit with me on the couch. He rubs my leg just as a heavy contraction comes.

"Breathe," he says. "Bubble of peace." This was a phrase used over and over in the HypnoBirthing class Sean and I had taken while I was pregnant with Finch. It was supposed to keep me grounded and in some high, new age state of meditative bliss while in labor. And despite the intention of getting me into some blissy groove, "bubble of peace" had instead become shorthand for funny shit you do when you can't imagine the fact that birthing your child can go sideways. The phrase evokes patchouli-scented rooms and banging drums and our naïveté. And in this moment, on the couch, whispering "bubble of peace," Sean *is* funny, and I do this hiccupy, gasping laugh.

Things have been tense between us since Seattle. When I picked him up at the airport after his trip, he slumped in the car. They'd barely slept, he complained. I must have been trying to kill him. It was, I told myself, a joke—but there'd been no shared *Ha ha*, no collective and intimate knowing, no warmth whatsoever. Since then I'd felt a cold anger for the fact that he'd never said thank you for the trip, never expressed any appreciation at all. I also felt guilt for wanting his appreciation in the first place, for knowing I'd given the gift to try to make up for the burden of my insomnia. I'd felt far from him and we'd moved around the house like strangers. But now, in the early-morning light, we're together—as together as we've been in months—and I'm amazed at how quickly the gap between us repairs.

"Will you call Hollis?"

"Yeah," he says. "Now?"

"Yes, I think so. Tell her we'll call her again when we get to the hospital. Tell her it'll be an hour, maybe."

And then it's 6:00 a.m. I'm beginning to gasp with each contraction and the sear that remains afterward. I'm not feeling quite so hot anymore, not so centered. I want to go to the hospital. Now. Where's Christina? We need to go. Sean calls again; she's just down the street, turning the corner. She'll be here. I don't remember this hurting so much. The fire started but it doesn't stop. My belly is tight as a drum, fisted and furious. And then Christina's here. She and Finch will be fine. We get into the car.

Sean drives down 500 South to I-15. Morning traffic's heavy. Sean tries to drive smoothly but a black Fiat cuts in front of him. He stomps on the brake and I cry out.

"Sorry," he says, looking over at me. "I'm sorry, he just—"

"It's okay," I say, my eyes closed. "Just please don't brake so hard."

"Sorry."

And then we're on the highway, surreal in our little spaceship moving toward the hospital that's so massive, people call it the Death Star. Cars pass us with people talking on their cell phones, hurrying to get to work on time, to punch in, to begin a normal day with normal watercooler chat. Sean brakes as a Chrysler hurtles toward an exit. I sit as motionless as I can. I close my eyes again. *Breathe.* My belly won't relax. Burning heat. Every movement now is pain, constant and relentless. I'm dizzy with it, my eyes locked shut to escape my body.

Finally, we're at the hospital. Sean pulls up for the valet. Thank God for valets. Oh, sweet mercy. A wheelchair arrives and I move like lead. Legs first, then pelvis. I'm down and Sean takes the handles. The seat is faux leather and flaking. I rub my fingertip over one of the flakes, tearing it, my finger burrowing into the synthetic fill. Past the entryway toward the main doors, a very pregnant twentysomething woman stands with her hands pressed against the glass. She's hunched and static, with her eyes closed. A young man hovers behind her, hand on her back, looking terrified.

Sean rolls me to the front counter and the slow litany of questions begins. He answers each one, tapping his finger, his leg jostling. Finally, I'm given a wrist bracelet and a nurse leads me to my room. She helps me put on a robe and then the belts around my stomach to monitor the contractions and our girl's heartbeat. She checks my dilation. Six centimeters.

"This is a VBAC, is that correct?" she asks Sean.

"A what?"

"Vaginal birth after cesarean," she explains, her eyebrows lifting slightly. "You're the father?"

"Oh, yeah. Yes. Sorry, I didn't know the name. Yes, we're trying for a natural birth. We have a nurse-midwife on the second floor or wherever their offices are."

Sean and the nurse talk for a while and I float in and out. Sean asks if I'm hungry. Do I need an egg biscuit? A fruit salad, maybe? Some cantaloupe balls? This is how he shows love. He'd make a prime rib dinner right there in the hospital room if he could. He'd whip sweet potatoes with butter and molasses and mold them into a ship. The nurse leaves and Sean calls Hollis again. She's getting dressed, she says. She'll be here in half an hour. Sean's hand is heavy on my shoulder. He asks me something but I've tunneled down. It hurts. My breath pulses in and out in fiery beats. My belly feels singularly numb and torched. The nurse comes back in. My contractions are close together and very strong. I should be dilated more. They're keeping a close eye on the baby's heartbeat, she says, and then I open my eyes.

"I want an epidural," I tell her. "As soon as possible."

"What?" Sean's confused. We've just gotten to the hospital and I've already blown my bubble of peace. I'm a natural-birthing failure.

And so the nurse, whose name is Taylor, calls the anesthesiologist and we're in luck, because he's between C-sections and can come right away. Taylor stays and watches the baby's heartbeat on the monitor. It's wavering just a bit, flagging after each contraction like someone who's been hit in the head with a rock and has a moment of disorientation before stumbling forward.

The anesthesiologist comes, and Hollis arrives, and then the hours start to float by. Sean and Hollis take turns sleeping and getting coffee. Hollis rubs my feet and my hands. She gives me the tea ice chips she promised to make.

It's late in the afternoon when the nurse-midwife is called. It isn't Angela. It's never Angela, and I've accepted the fact that someone I've likely met only once will deliver my baby. This nurse-midwife has neatly carved, yellowish hair and strong hands. Her name is Georgia, she says. Georgia from Salt Lake City. Born and bred. I remember her voice, low and loud as a football coach. *Hut hut!* She and I talked on the phone when my contractions were so bad, she recommended I come in for several fetal stress tests. Taylor and another nurse are also in the room. "We're getting ready," they tell me. The contractions are very close together. It's almost time to push.

I'm arranged into a half-reclining position with Georgia sitting neatly between my legs. Sean sits on a chair near my right shoulder. We're all prepared. The team has assembled but I'm still so far away.

Taylor's watching the monitor to pace the contractions. The epidural has numbed me to the extent I can't feel my body's signals to push. Taylor will act as my body's proxy by way of the monitor. She tells Sean to help me grab my legs. We're awkward and fumbling but we get my legs up. She counts down and when she says, "Push," I do my best imitation of pushing. I clench my face and imagine I'm contracting muscles that could, for all practical purposes, be in another state. I'm told to relax. Sean says something encouraging. Taylor counts down again, her brow furrowing as she looks at the monitor. "Push." We do this for an interminable amount of time. I keep hoping for some measure of progress—a lit face, Georgia standing with hands out and ready—but it feels as if we're all actors in a Sartre play, pushing and pushing, with no one exiting and nothing happening at all.

After what feels like hours, a man in scrubs walks in. He's intent, with none of the quiet caution of the residents or nurses. He has a brief discussion with Taylor before coming to the bedside.

"Ms. Bond," he says, all business. "I'm Dr. Katz, head of OB-GYN for the hospital. We've been watching your child's heartbeat on our main system of monitors. She hasn't been recovering well and it's serious enough that you need to consider a C-section. I know you wanted to have a VBAC, but I think it's unwise at this point."

I look down at Georgia and up at Sean. I can't believe this is happening. Georgia's glaring hard at Dr. Katz, her hands in a state of suspended animation in front of her, as if the baby were sliding out this very second.

"This baby's at a two plus," Georgia shouts, furious, referring to the fact that my girl's head has descended into the birth canal. This means they'll have to pull her little head out of my pelvis because she's partway out the door. I find this a terrible idea.

"Can we have more time?" I ask.

"A little more," Dr. Katz says. "But we're keeping an eye on the baby."

Minutes later, in a haze of pushing but not pushing, I see a man in white come in the door. He walks to my right side and Sean, Georgia, and I watch with horror as he inserts a large needle into the catheter taped to my arm.

"Just getting you prepped," he says to me, and his voice sounds slowed down, like an old record with a finger tracking it, the voice growing deeper as it slows to a stop.

"What the hell are you doing?" Georgia yells at the man, her eyes wide.

"I was told to prep Ms. Bond for a C-section," the man in white says, confused, his hand still attached to the needle in my arm.

"We did not give the go-ahead," Georgia snaps. She's pissed. "This baby *does not* need to come via C-section."

"Dr. Katz told me to prep her," the man says, backing out of the room.

And then it's a wash. The anesthetic's quick, and within minutes I can't move my body at all. "Push," Taylor says, but my body's gone icy and numb, and before we know it, there's a rush of people in blue scrubs and we're out the door with a resident running alongside. I've heard the qualifiers before: "You must know the risks—uterine laceration, bowel laceration, any and all manner of laceration, hemorrhage, death." Yes. Quite. And here we are. The operating room. Another faltering heart. Another C-section.

I'm hefted like a small whale onto the open deck of the operating table and laid out, arms at my sides, mouth dry as bone. I'm cleaned and shaved to the skin by people who move around me like I'm a specimen, a large, heaving specimen whose baby is faltering and whom they must slice open soon, pull out the child, save the shrinking heart. The female resident exchanges jokes with Dr. Katz. She's wearing a kerchief over her hair, not a puffball cinched with elastic. The resident looks over the sheet placed between my head and body.

"Do you feel this?" She pokes a needle somewhere.

"No."

"This?" She moves her arm.

"No."

I can barely form the word. My mouth is a desert camp in Dubai. And then Sean arrives, scrubbed and clothed in pants and shirt and puffball hat, all of that filmy material, nearly gossamer but likely made of sad, dead trees, the leftover pulp that wasn't suitable for anything but this throwaway medical attire designed to keep hair and germs out of the sterile rooms, to stave off infection and death. Sean settles himself next to my head, but I can't see him because I'm immobile now, pinned down like a butterfly in a glass case, and we're all hushed because it's nearly time. I'll be gutted, my uterus lifted out of my body and onto my chest, intestines hanging, the pool of my pelvis open and surging with blood.

And they begin cutting. I'm so deep down in my body, I can't even feel my baby. *Get her out. Cut me open at the base, tear my root from its source.* And they do. Dr. Katz is on my left, the female resident on my right, and the layers of skin give way easily until they don't—suddenly they don't because a layer of adhesions from the first C-section has woven my uterus up and into the muscles of my abdomen. And yes, this is a problem; this is a mighty problem . . .

Dr. Katz says "Fuck" under his breath and raises his arm up, above my body, scalpel to the sky. Later, the female resident told us she felt a flutter in her stomach, because this was something she hadn't seen, the uterus so glued to the muscles, there was nothing to do but shave off layers of the abdomen with a razor. My God, the female resident said, she thought she might be sick with all the blood, the abdomen contracting like a thrashing animal, the blood so thick and pooling.

And it takes so long. Sean sits and then decides to stand. He takes several pictures of the meat and blood, my body like raw steak, like a cut cow. It's impossible for me to fathom why he does this. It's as if my cut and bleeding body is simply a novelty, a fascinating vista from a new mountain instead of the hemorrhaging body that is his wife and baby on the table. Later, when he shows me the digital images, I recoil, horrified. He deletes the pictures from his camera so fast I wonder if he'll even remember that it happened. But the photos lodge in my memory along with a deep sense of betrayal for which I have no words.

The process of separating my uterus from my abdomen is delicate. Both are becoming mangled, but Dr. Katz is intent and finally my uterus lets go, and it's lifted out and opened and our girl is there, alive. They haul her like a fish into the boat of the living, her blue eyes wide, shining in her pearl-blue body, awake as if we had startled her out of her deep-ocean sleep.

And then they attend to her and there's an attempt to reassemble my body. Intestines are tucked back into my pelvis and my uterus is sewn up and similarly placed, but there's still so much blood. Dr. Katz stands, his hands pressed against my uterus and abdomen. The female resident, too, attempts to stop the blood, and a slow creep of cold begins moving into my arms and legs.

Dr. Katz clears his throat. He leans over the little blue curtain separating me from the rest of my body and tells me they may have to perform a hysterectomy to save my life. His tone is neither soft nor hard but practical, as if he's telling me there are no shoes of this kind in my size; perhaps I should try the boots, the brown ones with a slight heel. There's an exchange between Dr. Katz and another doctor who's been in the room but who I can't see. They tell a joke of some kind entirely unrelated to my body or the blood that's making a furious lake inside of me. They laugh and then discuss the relative merits of different types of matrixed material designed to aid in efforts such as theirs. There's an agreement to try one of the materials and the material is procured and then placed inside the gaping hole that is my abdomen.

And through all this the cold comes like something whispered into my body. They show me our girl again and I notice she looks like the Egyptian goddess Nefertiti, the back of her head elegant and long and strange, the bones of the cranium suctioned and molded by the birth canal. Sean takes her and soon I'm told I'll keep my uterus, that the matrix fiber has worked to stop the hemorrhaging. The female resident and a nurse work to pull my body together and place staples through my skin. I feel tugs: the two of them on either side of me, grappling with the slip of skin and blood, the layers of meat that have yawned open and do not easily refold over the bulk of my intestines.

And then I'm brought out of the operating room and into a recovery room. There are machines everywhere and I can hear my heartbeat pinging mechanically through the room. Taylor's there. She'll take care of me, she says; everything'll be fine. "I'm so cold," I tell her, and she brings warmed blankets, but I'm still so cold, arctic and heavy and beginning to shake. Taylor stands, watching a monitor intensely, and she has a tiny microphone attached to the pocket of her scrubs. She talks to someone, her brow tight, her eyes flicking back and forth over the screen.

It's cold. It's so fucking cold. I'm beginning to shake hard now, like someone naked on an icy road in a Minnesota snowstorm. I'm shaking so hard, my neck muscles cramp. My head rolls back and forth like a metronome to loosen the throttle that's taken my neck and body. Something dark hovers in the corner. It's leaning in. It's watching me.

The sound of my heartbeat reverberates around the room and then Taylor begins yelling into her microphone for blood. She wants blood *stat*, she shouts, and I rock my head back and forth, listening to my heart counted out in beats. Taylor yells numbers into the microphone. My blood pressure's falling, she yells. We need blood and my God it's a misery of cold and I can't stop shaking, can't brace myself against the freeze that's entered my body, the shadow that's moving in from the corner, reaching for me.

Scrubbed bodies rush around the room. I'm pumped full of blood and fluids and still my blood pressure drops. Rupture. Blood a still, ruby lake. Sound thunders in the room. Hush. Someone tucks more heated blankets on my body. I rock my head back and forth; I'm given morphine to combat the pain. My heart thrums slowly through the machine. I listen to the *ping ping ping ping* getting slower and slower until it stops. It's like a ball bouncing loudly in a room until gravity presses its thumb *down*.

And I hang there, in that space between beats, listening for my heart to start. My body's a nub, a nothing. I don't know where our girl has been taken. She's in another room with another person, walls of waiting between us. I float. I wonder if I'll see her again. Will I see my Nefertiti girl, or will she be motherless, raised by Sean and his sisters and always with the story that her mother died in childbirth, that she never knew her, never once saw her face, only saw her in pictures and stories and the occasional dream. I wonder if this is how I'll die: freezing cold, listening for my heartbeat, and wanting only to see my daughter's face. *Let me look at her face. That pearl body. Please. Don't let me die yet. I'm not ready to go. Don't let darkness lift me out. Let me see my beautiful girl just one more time.*

# SPECIMEN HAZE

*November 2009*

AFTER SEVEN HOURS IN THE POST-OP room, I stabilize, and nurses roll my bed into my very own hospital suite. The room has an expanse of white linoleum, a tan Barcalounger, and a window seat that doubles as a small bed. I stay on the hospital bed, hooked up to IVs, my stomach high and puffy. My face and body are bloated unrecognizably from all the fluids that were pumped into me. My fingers and toes resemble a bouquet of sausages. I'm told my body won't remain troll-like for longer than a week—two at most.

Hollis and Sean stay in the room with me, and when they bring Chloe in, she latches on immediately. Chloe. That's what we've decided to call her. It's an elegant, old-fashioned name; a name like velvet. I rub my fingertips over her long head, cup my hand under her legs and back, her body a little comma in the crook of my arm. Chloe. I nurse her, ecstatic, hopped up on the warmth of being alive. I fall asleep while she's nursing and wake only a little when her head rolls to the side. Sean takes her and holds her body next to his chest. His face is lit and calm and beautiful. Then sleep comes and it's the best thing in the world. It's warm and dreamless and I don't wake again until the sky's inky black and a nurse is hovering over my body, checking my vitals and incision.

Then Chloe needs to eat again and it's heaven, my body with her body, her head heavy in my hand, eyes fluttering shut with the night.

After four days, Chloe and I are discharged. Sean has been going back and forth, working during the days while Christina watches Finch. He visits at night when Christina can stay late with our boy. I'm told to take ibuprofen and Percocet every four hours for the pain. *Contact the doctor if my uterus starts to bleed. Don't pick up anything over five pounds. Don't walk too much. And the swelling's uncomfortable, yes, but it will go down. Put your feet up. Sleep when you can. Take it easy.*

Finch doesn't understand why I can't pick him up. He looks at me with pleading eyes, arms held out, and I tell him Mama can't pick him up because her stomach has been turned inside out. Sean picks Finch up and nuzzles him. We try lying on the bed together while I nurse Chloe but Finch crawls over to my stomach. Sean grabs him as I wince. I'm ten pounds heavier than when I entered the hospital and my belly's still springy and inflated. I could paint it red and draw a clown face and I'd be my own personal bounce house.

AFTER A DREAM of seven nights blending into days, Sean's mom, Sharon, comes to stay with us. She lives in Idaho and usually stays with Sean's sister, who lives about twenty minutes from us, but with my being so cut up and compromised, she's here. It's difficult for Sean. Something happens when his mom's around; some wound that's never closed pulses with anger. He tries to keep a lid on it, but clamping down just makes things worse. All Sharon wants to do is help. She lives for God and her children but something about her endless and hungry banter is, for Sean, like being forced into a locked and windowless room.

Sharon tackles the laundry, which is no small task. Who knew you could go through so many onesies in a day? She scrubs the kitchen counters to a bright sheen and organizes and puts things into neat little piles. Sean tells her not to move things. "Sorry," Sharon says, moving the pile to the right. He hates when she moves things. "Sorry, sorry," she says, moving the pile to the left. There'll be a momentary hush. Sharon will suck her breath in and her hand will hover in the air, eyes darting back and forth before she resumes her banter. There's so much to do, she says. How's his friend—the one who got divorced and then disappeared for a while? Was he drinking? Was he on medication? She's changed her medication, she tells us. It keeps her from crying. If she starts crying, she says, scrubbing the white tile counter, she doesn't think she'll be able to stop. Sean stands in the kitchen for a moment, his eyes hard and motionless. "Can you just not talk for one minute?" he says. "Just one minute?" Sharon sucks in her lips as if she's been slapped. Sean leaves for Home Depot and doesn't return until the sun's gone down.

Sharon takes my list and goes to the grocery store. Afterward she makes a valiant effort to teach Finch some block-stacking maneuvers in the front room. Blocks crash to the floor repeatedly. "Sorry," Sharon yells from the living room. "Are you asleep?" I'm on the bed with Chloe. I rest—or pretend at rest. I stopped taking the Ambien CR after Chloe was born, sure that my hormonal imbalance would right itself, but sleep remains so terribly thin. "It's okay," I tell her. "Don't worry, we're just lying here."

At night, stretched out on the couch in the front room, blankets piled over her head, Sharon reads her Bible and plays solitaire on her iPad. Sean claims she'd sleep on a bed of nails if that's what was offered. And this somehow makes him angrier, makes him want to offer her a bed of nails in the basement with the heat turned off.

A few days into her visit, Sharon tells me the Bible says one must not incite one's children to anger. I tell her Sean's anger isn't her responsibility, but this distresses her. There are so many raw spots between them. I try to create gentleness and comfort in the house. I know I'm overcompensating for Sean's anger, but Sharon is like a nervous, frightened animal. I tell her how grateful I am for her help. She talks to me about God and her medications and her relationship with Sean's father, which ended savagely. Sean remembers a time when he was eight or nine, just before their divorce, when his dad was mocking Sharon about something. They were in the kitchen. She was making dinner and his smiling humor was cruel and indirect and Sharon got so upset, she started to bang her head against the cabinets. Sean's dad laughed. At one point Sharon took an entire bag of sugar and dumped it on top of Sean's dad's head.

After four days of Sharon being at our house, Sean can't take it. He sends her to stay with his sister. This is how it often goes. Sharon gets shuttled between houses, people calling her for help and then sending her away. The whole thing makes me horribly sad and Sean stays angry and shut away for days, the wound so big I can barely get near him.

FOR TWO WEEKS Chloe's a beatific, warm little lump I carry around. Then she wakes to the world; her face pinches up and she cries the kind of cry that has no end. I try nursing, I try putting her in the swing. I try cooing and jostling. Nothing. She howls and there's nothing I can do to soothe her. When she first came home, Sean and I made a little nest for her in the closet at the foot of our bed. We reasoned she'd be comfortable and close and Finch wouldn't hear her cries at night. After a few nights of this, we make a desperate change in the configuration. Chloe is up four or five times every night to nurse and often falls asleep just as Finch is waking up to the day. Sean decides to sleep downstairs on a blow-up mattress and I'll stay in the bed to co-sleep with Chloe. I tell myself I knew having two infants would be hard. *It will get better. Sleep will come. This is a normal mama tunnel. People do it all the time, all the time, all the time. Just hang on.*

During the day, Sean and I develop a desperate strategy of musical baby. We take turns swapping Chloe between a front carrier, the little rocker that fits on the kitchen table, and the double stroller. The double stroller is used only when one of us starts to redline, which, as we know from the DVDs given to us by the hospital, can lead one to unthinkable acts. After what feels like hours of her wailing, I bundle Finch and Chloe, give each of them a bottle, and push the stroller as fast as I can—once, twice, three times around the block—bouncing over frozen ridges of snow and ice.

Most Saturdays, Sean leaves for much of the day. There are errands and hikes, there is sod to drop off, and there are people to meet. I'm hammered with exhaustion. Finch and Chloe are typically to bed by 7:30 p.m. and up by 5:30 a.m. By 11:00 a.m. I've strolled and bounced and swung Chloe. She quiets for a few moments, but the minute motion stops, all hell breaks loose. Finally, I put her in the front carrier, bounce with vigorous fury on our yellow yoga ball, and read her the first three chapters of Michael Cunningham's book *Specimen Days*. It's brilliant. Finch crashes out on the couch and Chloe slips into a happy baby trance. It's this moment that I fall deeply in love with Michael Cunningham. Who knew Cunningham's beautiful words and plays on Walt Whitman had the power to transfix infants and their desperate mothers? There are innumerable ways to survive a colicky baby, and Michael Cunningham is mine. I spend the next month bouncing on that yoga ball, Chloe tucked into the carrier that cradles her against my chest, as I read through the book. Later, I move on to *The Lord of the Rings*. I survive the days in this way. It's the nights that again become alien.

Delivering Chloe doesn't deliver me from the insomnia. Three weeks after Chloe is born, night becomes a hole, a tear in the fabric that won't mend. After feeding Chloe at night, I don't fall back asleep. *Tick tick tick* goes the clock in my head. I bounce Chloe during the day and at night my eyes remain pinned open to the darkness. Soon I begin to think about the pills. Night after night I think of them. They will help me sleep. This is all I want. I pray every night that something in my body will loosen and sleep will become normal again. Wasn't it supposed to normalize after the baby was born? I feel a growing desperation. There's a bottle of Ambien in the bathroom. *Just one*, I think. *Just tonight, so I can sleep.* Then: *Don't be ridiculous. My body will return to normal eventually. I will do my meditations and my valerian tea*, I tell myself. *I will be strong. I will not take the fucking pills.*

# SLIP 'N' SLIDE

*December 2009*

CHLOE'S ASLEEP. IT'S 2:00 A.M. AND I've been watching her for hours. The anxiety about not sleeping is relentless. I try meditating. I try listing all the states and their capitals. If Chloe would just wake up, I could feed her and get the wash of relaxing mama hormones. It'd be something. Instead, I get up. I shuffle to the bathroom, flick the light on, and stare at my bottle of little blue pills. I have half a bottle left. I'd planned on throwing it away after delivering Chloe, but I never did. I left it there like insurance.

The light in the bathroom is a bulb with a frosted-glass lily over it. We have a series of shelves in front of the toilet that Sean cut into the wall. He's never really finished the job, never put in wood to line the edges, and I imagine splinters jutting out at every angle. My bottle's on the third shelf, tucked behind the Tylenol. *I'm taking one*, I think. I've got to sleep. Something's wrong with me. Sleep is the currency for which I'd trade anything. It's crushing, this nerve-stripped feeling, and it's here again every day. I'll take the Ambien CR—just tonight. Just for now. Maybe one every other night. I'll try herbs on the others.

Valerian, skullcap. Maybe melatonin. I'll be strong. But tonight I can't. Tonight I need a pill.

THE NEXT MORNING Sean sits at the kitchen table, watching Stephen Colbert videos on the computer. I wake after having watched Chloe for at least four hours and wandering the front room for two. I'd hoped having Chloe close would help me sleep. *Anything. Jesus.* It helps some nights. Other nights I lie in bed and think about the pills. *Did I take one the night before? Did I imagine that?*

Finch sits in front of the toy basket, pulling the toys out and hurling them against the floor. This cracks him up. Each toy is a new delight—a Woody doll, a fist-sized bulldozer, a Hug Me puppy. *My God!* I imagine him thinking. *These things actually fly; they bounce!* He's the child I love the most right now. I know I'm not supposed to say this—that I love one child better than the other. But Finch is a soft, Lucretian atom; he's butter. His arms grip my neck and he wraps himself around me like a little koala, and in those instants the world is beautiful.

Chloe's a developing larva and I don't love her yet. I'm supposed to love her, to be transfixed, but I don't. I'm not. She thrashes and refuses to be put down. The howling starts the minute we lay her on the bed or on the soft baby blanket in the front room with the glittery mobile rotating over her head. The girl has to be in motion. I've taken to bringing her baby swing into the bathroom so I can take showers. With the thrum of water, she's quiet, but the second I turn it off, there's a brief silence—a stunned pause—and then her howls beat the walls of the house.

Days stream together. I saw Ivy just after Chloe was born but it's been hard to stay connected. She returned from Alaska and was offered a job at an online university. She's busy, and every day I feel buried. And now snow obscures everything—sky the color of snow, one long wash of white. Chloe woke the previous night at midnight, then one o'clock, then two. I finally rolled over and fed her, those round eyes staring at me, at the ceiling, staring from some other place—not quite here, not quite there. Larval. Wailing, unless I walk. Wailing unless I shower, letting water drum on tiles. Wailing unless I bounce on the yoga ball, reading to her from *The Lord of the Rings*.

Sean gets desperate and buys a television for the room downstairs. He's working through his shifts with Chloe by watching episodes of *Battlestar Galactica*. He walks small circles in front of the air mattress, bouncing her in the carrier. The night before last, she refused to sleep. I brought her down at 1:00 a.m. and she and Sean watched the Cylons lay waste to a colony of humans. As the sun came up, there were tracks in the carpet in front of the television. Chloe finally fell asleep as the battlestar *Galactica* surged through space in search of a fabled refuge known as Earth. "It was epic," Sean tells me, his eyes heavy and listless. "It was fucking epic."

That Christmas, my mother comes from California, and Sean and I practically dump Chloe into her arms. "Jostling works," we tell her, "and she loves the front carrier. Just don't stop moving."

My mother stays at a motel one block away. Sean and I don't have a spare bed, and while his mother will sleep on the couch or the floor, my mother will not. She's happy with the motel and the bad coffee, she tells us. She doesn't mind walking the block through winter slush the color of charcoal.

After weeks of being inside and the blur of night and day, Sean and I are in a stupor. We get a small tree and make efforts at holiday cheer. *Look!* I imagine saying to Finch and Chloe. *A tree with shiny, pretty things! We are symbolic in this household! We celebrate life in the midst of an interminable winter! Salutations to Jesus Christ, Mary, and all the wise ones throughout history. Salutations to the Jews and Muslims and Hindus! We embrace equal opportunity spirituality in this household, and we love trees!*

My mother isn't a cleaner. She helps with the dishes and jiggles Chloe until Chloe wails, which most often means Chloe wants a different brand of jiggling, a shift to the right or left, a slight jog through the house or around the block. I take Chloe from her. Sean makes a roast and I ask my mother if she'd like some tea.

When I was young, I saw my mother's sadness and anger as something that was somehow my fault. My brother, Chris, and I never knew what to expect from one day to the next, so we adapted. My brother shut himself away from her and kept his door closed. I became the nurturer, the fixer, the diplomat. I had to deny my own feelings of sadness, fear, and anger in order to survive. I was constantly walking on eggshells, serving tea, afraid of the fire that could erupt in her that would burn down our house.

My mother would hold in the fire and rage until she couldn't, and it would rise up and she would become someone I didn't recognize. I remember being five or six in our little duplex. It was a Saturday and I'd done something intolerable. Perhaps I'd gotten up early. Perhaps I'd tried to cook an egg. We were in the kitchen. She screamed, and my little body felt weighted, pinned against the cabinets. My brother ran upstairs and I was there alone with a rage that had no beginning and no end. I was a bad child. I was ungrateful. She couldn't stand being a mother. She had no help. No one. Finally, after what felt like a lifetime of my clutching the rim of the cabinets behind me, eyes wide with terror, she sucked her rage in. She made a slow, silent retreat to her bedroom. She shut the door and didn't come out for days.

During these times, Chris and I would watch TV in the room next to hers. After several days she'd come out, limp as dough. We'd all sit together watching cartoons until she could get up and fix dinner. Later she'd be raw with guilt that would bring a nameless, awkward tenderness. We'd pretend. We'd hope it wouldn't happen again.

Something inside me fractured during her furies. It was inside of that broken place that I started writing poetry. It became my enchanted castle, my refuge, my heart. I sewed words around me like a quilt. I survived being broken and mother-lost in this way. I held the bleeding parts inside me with words, and the words were kind and they were mine.

Now Mom and I sit on the couch and watch a cloud of sparrows dip and sway in the sky outside the window. "Look," I say to Chloe, who's firmly latched on to my breast, "can you see the birds outside? Can you see the way they move like water?"

Mom holds a cup of black coffee. She's been telling me about work. After rehab, she worked her way up to becoming one of the most successful executive recruiters in Silicon Valley. This lasted for two decades, at which point she decided to leave it all behind and open a pet boutique. This was years ago. She took the mint she'd made and opened iPaw, a store with bling enough to satisfy Paris Hilton and monthly fashion shows where leggy women walked dogs with sapphire collars down a carpeted runway.

There was just one problem: my mother had no idea how to run a small business. The recession hit and she spent and kept spending, filling her store with more bling, more doggie beds shaped like Rolls-Royces, more dog-sized ball gowns and tuxedos. She was nouveau riche and stumbling. When a man named Johnny Ocean came in—a man resembling a blood sausage in a crisp Armani suit—she was done for. Johnny Ocean promised to help her with advertising, with market saturation, with finances to help keep her business going. All she needed to do was buy into his secret network and the world would be hers. Cashier's checks were purchased. Promises sparkled and evaporated. Johnny Ocean was my mother's Madoff. Within a year, he had disappeared and my mother had lost everything.

She returned to her career as a recruiter, but she'd lost her connections and the market had grown soft. She now lives in a two-room apartment near the freeway—barely enough for her and her three dogs.

"I'm getting enough work to survive," she tells me. "But I don't go out to eat. I don't buy new clothes." She sighs and stares down at Chloe, who's beginning to look like a drunken sailor.

"You did the best you could."

"I didn't listen to you. I didn't listen to anybody. I just kept spending and spending." She stares out the window. "Anyway, this trip isn't about me." She pats my leg. "When are we going to open the presents?"

Sean walks in with coffee and Finch. The two of them have just gotten up and Finch stuns us with his steady stream of yabba dabba talk punctuated with "Ohs" and wide, startled eyes. Sean's sleepy and shirtless, wearing rumpled flannel pajama bottoms. He drops onto the couch next to me.

I can't pinpoint when the wall between us came up, when it began to feel like there was so little left between Sean and me. It's more than just the stress of two infants and my insomnia. Something hard and angry stalks the shadows between us. All warmth evaporates into a cold silence broken open only by us discussing logistics: When will he be back? Do we need diapers? Has Finch said anything new? His body stays but he's emotionally gone, his eyes often taking on a glazed quality as he projects himself anywhere but here. He often has the look of someone stoned but aware that an unfortunate byproduct of being stoned is the proclivity to drift—one's attention at once vaporous and dreamy, paranoid and hyper-focused.

As I've done with my mother, I take his anger and retreat inward. I try to transform it. If *I* can get better, *we'll* be better. If I can only be kinder, his eyes will once again enliven and look at me with warmth. We're toxic—him leaning away and me riddled with a guilt that's my way of trying to control a loss I don't understand.

"Merry Christmas," he says, kissing my cheek. He toasts my mom with his cup of coffee.

"Merry Christmas," I say, touching his muscled chest. Despite the wall between us, I still feel a crush when he's shirtless and close. The insomnia has its teeth in me, and I struggle nightly with the pills, but the heat still comes. It's Christmas, I think. There's the slightest bit of softness in his demeanor. I don't know where the edge has gone or when it will come back, but in this moment, this little bit of soft is enough.

We open presents, trying to teach Finch how to tear paper. His fine motor skills are still awkward, so we rip and throw the paper for him. He gets cars, a small blue guitar, and Play-Doh. Sean and I exchange massage certificates to a fancy Japanese spa. And for my mother: a turquoise sweater to match her eyes.

Later, Sean cooks steaks while Mom tries to teach Finch how to hold his guitar. I feel warm and safe for the first time in months. When I walk into the kitchen after getting Chloe down for her nap, Sean wraps his long arms around me and pulls me in. This shock of tenderness unravels me. My God, I've missed him so much. I sink into his body. Fingers trace the outline of my shoulder blades and slide to my lower back. He presses his hips gently into mine. Heat. It's still there—even in my dead-tired body, even with the wall that will continue to rise between us. I can't believe it, but it's still there. Heat. Merry Christmas.

MY PILLS ARE running out. Christmas warmth has come and gone and now a January cold settles in. I haven't wanted to take the leftover pills at all, but now that I am, I promise myself this will be it. There will be no new prescription, no new bottle to sit on the bathroom counter. I've always hated pills. To get more feels like some kind of personal failure, and still, every night I count them. I have seventeen left and then ten. I promise myself I won't take one for two nights. I need to save them for if it gets really bad, but I'm taking them every third night now and scratching at the walls the other two. What will I do when I run out? Anxiety lives like a stranger in my body. I fight myself daily, sure the anxiety comes from the fatigue and overwhelm of caring for two infants. I don't need the pills, I tell myself. What I need is to be stronger.

# STAGE OF THE BARGAIN

*January 2010*

ONE MORNING IN JANUARY, SEAN SITS at the kitchen table with his coffee and laptop. He reads the HuffPost and the *Los Angeles Times*. He looks at Facebook. It's fascinating, what all these Facebook people are doing. So many vacations and friends! Ski trips to Canada, walking on cooled lava in Hawaii! Pictures of glowing families with glowing backgrounds—a little boy smiling up at his mother; the mother, model-like with perfect jeans and soft, petaled lips, looking down. Such lives of leisure and beauty!

He closes the laptop and tells me he needs to ski. He needs to get out. Yes, I say, neither of us is getting out and we need it. We need to fill our joy pockets. We've just had a night of snowfall. Chloe sleeps on the bed and Finch pushes the buttons on his Hug Me puppy and Sean gathers his things: skis, poles, a backpack filled with Clif Bars and sandwiches, water and hot chocolate, his stash of pot. He leaves after swearing he won't be gone long, that he'll take the kids for a drive when he gets back so I can try to sleep. This is his negotiation. He'll look away from what he's determined is my pathology. He'll do it, he says with no emotion, "to give me a break."

The door shuts.

I throw in a load of laundry and wash the dishes.

An hour passes, then two, then three.

I nurse and jostle Chloe. I crawl on the floor with the two of them, trying to show Chloe the magic of getting on all fours. She's just turned three months old and she no longer howls to be held. I look into those honey eyes and a well of love opens up in me. I make smacking noises in her ear and she falls over with giggles, leaning her warm head into my face. We stay like that, nuzzling, until she decides she must get up and track down the Hug Me puppy. It's too cold to do anything outside, so we play with cars and blocks. Finch wrestles Chloe until she wails, and I separate them. The hours stretch on like an endless road.

I feel eclipsed with guilt for not being the shining mother. And Sean has become edgy with resentment. Two days ago he drove the kids to Tooele and back—an hour drive. When he walked in the door, holding Chloe in his arms, he said he'd decided that taking the kids for drives so I could rest was enabling me, as if my persistent insomnia were some kind of dysfunctional behavior. He put Chloe down, kissed her head, and went back to get Finch out of the car. When he returned, with Finch in his car seat, he continued as if we'd had no break in the conversation at all. He'd thought a lot about it, he said. He was worried about this *enabling*. He didn't want to do it. He wouldn't. My jaw dropped. I felt like someone had thrown a bowling ball at my chest.

Four hours go by. Sean is not back. I start arguing with myself. I cry for five minutes in the bathroom. I'm not Donna Reed. I don't shine. It's all so fucked-up.

I tell myself I won't be my mother. I won't hurt the people I love with my fury. So I do what I've always done. I overcompensate by becoming hyperrational. At least, I imagine I'm hyperrational, but I'm really a sleep-deprived rage machine. I'm in the kitchen, washing dishes, when the internal argument really heats up. Finch is asleep downstairs and Chloe is in the little rocker that I've set up on the kitchen table. I stare at the peeling yellow linoleum of the kitchen floor, the grime between the kitchen tiles. I can't stand the filth of this place. There's nowhere to run and it's just me and my wobbly head and two infants. I slam a cabinet and stomp to the front room to look out the window. No Sean. Never Sean. I stare at the milk stain on the front-room rug and then it's just a shit show with the two parts of me grappling like wrestlers in the room in my head.

The argument goes something like this:

You've got to be more understanding.

*Yeah, I understand that he's a complete asshole.*

Well, maybe not an asshole. He's bringing home the bacon now and that's not easy. He's got to be terrified. I mean, try to walk in his shoes . . .

*I'd like to see him take care of two infants after getting an hour of sleep. I'd like to see him walk in those shoes for a couple of months.*

You know how overwhelmed he gets. It's a lot of pressure.

*Poor bunny needs to take care of himself.*

He's doing his best . . .

*I hate him. He's been skiing for hours. What father of two infants does that? Four hours and no call, no "I'll be back soon, honey."*

It's hard for both—

*He sucks as a husband. He chews with his mouth open and warmth is just a precursor for putting his cock somewhere.*

You're not being fair. He's trying. You're both—

*Trying, my ass. He just wants some Betty Crocker chick with a surfer ass who'll do his laundry while he skis and who'll twinkle brightly over the pot roast when he gets home.*

Come on. Who doesn't want a Betty Crocker surfer chick? Who doesn't want some nice ass with their laundry?

*Fuck him.*

Be reasonable.

*Have I said that?*

Don't—

*Fuck him AND his cock AND his pot.*

So, hours later, when Sean gets home, we begin bargaining. We're at that stage. We agree that Sean will ski once or twice a week, and when he gets home, I'll get an hour to write. We'll schedule dates and sex. We have children and time is limited. We'll get a sitter to take the kids to the Discovery Gateway Children's Museum. We'll pay her so we can have sex in peace. Other days, we'll trade time. We'll clock in and out. We'll be adults.

EVERY DAY I watch for signs that Finch will speak. He's nineteen months old. I point up, say, "Light." Finch grabs my fingers and puts them in his mouth. He looks up. He does not say, "Light."

I fill a spoon with pureed mango and banana. Finch throws his arms into the air, palms wide and facing out. "Hooray!" I shout. "Field goal!" His blue eyes watch my mouth. He doesn't say any of these words. He laughs, tilts his head to the side, and leans forward to wrap his arms around my neck. Those arms.

"Hug," I say. "Mama. Papa. Hug."

He hugs. He says nothing.

I SPEND ALL month trying to read bits of David Foster Wallace's massive doorstop book *Infinite Jest* while in the bathroom. I have loved this man from afar for his brilliance, his dark and acrobatic wit on the page. I have read his work and wept at his bright and glorious brain, at the scalpel of his intelligence. And now I'm reading him in the bathroom. I take him in like little breaths because I need him alongside me now. I need his brilliance and his ache. Finch was three months old when Wallace committed suicide. I held Finch and cried when I found out. I felt lost-eyed, child things. Wallace had struggled with depression most of his life, and when his medication worked and then didn't, the crush of darkness took him and he couldn't go on. I can't help thinking that the tool of his intelligence, the thing that helped him divide, evaluate, and understand the world, also made it too heavy and ugly for him to bear. I wonder at the wisdom of holding this kind of intelligence up as our most prized accomplishment. I'm beginning to understand that Finch has a very different kind of intelligence, coming from a different expanse of perception—a blissful response to the air; an absolute rapture at the small things that create and ornament this life.

I haven't gotten far with *Infinite Jest*, but it doesn't matter. Wallace's words are air and I am breathing them in.

One month into my *Infinite Jest* breathing, I write a poem that's a love song to my boy and to David Foster Wallace. If only I could have introduced them. If only I could have given Wallace the kind of brilliance Finch lives with in every moment. *Look*, I'd say to Wallace, *this is what it's like when Beauty is everything you see.*

# INTO THE SOFT AIR

*February 2010*

I'm DOWN TO FOUR PILLS. I took an Ambien last night, but it was useless. It did nothing. I slept for three hours. And now it's my writing time and Christina has the kiddos. I left her watching *The Ellen DeGeneres Show*, Chloe asleep in her arms, Finch in the laundry room trying to figure out how to heft his body into the washing machine. Every time I leave, there's guilt. Every time I leave, there's relief.

My pants don't fit the way they used to. My belly has become softer and rounder, everything softer and rounder. My skin is dry. There are lines around my eyes, caused less from the babes than from the chronic sleep deprivation. I barely shower, opting to tie my hair into a knot at the top of my head. I've forgotten the act of wearing stylish jeans and boots.

With two kids, I'm lucky to brush my teeth. Lucky to pee. I've heard about this from other parents, heard about the impossibility of showers, the chaos of onesies, the desperate trips to the ER for snot sucking or concussive checks after a fall. I said, "Yes, yes—parenthood is hard." But mine were the comments of the uninitiated. I hadn't yet run to the ER at three in the morning because my boy couldn't breathe. I hadn't watched my life crumple under the weight of an identity I wasn't sure I could inhabit. I hadn't spent night after night walking my children through the halls to get them to sleep. I hadn't watched them sleep while the sun rose in front of me. My comments were pretentious and condescending and naïve. Hardy har har.

I'm Wifey now. I'm Mama. I'm she of the soup ladle, the scrub brush, and the backside. I'm the one called Night Walker. All my sheen has been worn away. I'm liquid. I'm on the floor.


I GET AN email telling me that a friend of mine has died. John. We were close for a short and intense period before I got together with Sean. We'd met at a party. It was summer, and the night was electric blue and John and I talked on the porch swing for three hours. He brought me gin and tonics with extra lime, long legs striding into the house and then out again to sit with me. At midnight, he convinced me to go on a bike tour of downtown Salt Lake City in search of gargoyles. We found six, looming high in the sky on Main Street and then on the Cathedral of the Madeleine, their bodies hunched like stone vultures.

Our friendship lasted five months. During that time, he was beautiful and euphoric. Joy was a fountain and we were the fountainheads. He was magnetic and tragic, and his intensity burned with a heat I knew couldn't last. We'd lie on the floor of his studio and listen to Bach and Radiohead and the Shins and sometimes we'd dance. Friends thought we were lovers, but the heat between us existed in the tension of longing that a physical relationship would have destroyed. We were twin flames burning hot, side by side, and staring into the dark. John burned like David Foster Wallace and I let myself burn with him. We shared a passion for music and late-night bike rides and John loved to surprise me with little samples of Malbec or Grenache wines, telling me I could taste the pepper or cherry on the back of my tongue if I closed my eyes. "Give into it," he'd say. "There's a Leonard Cohen afterlife if you watch for it." And I would and there it would be—raspberry, spice, an eternal sigh of sweet cherries.

John disappeared several weeks after I met Sean. He stopped calling and his number changed. I couldn't find him, and the hurt was burned away by the new heat with Sean. It wouldn't have been the same anyway. Sean was jealous. I let John go. Later, I heard his depression had surged. He was taking pills. I had no idea what kind. A friend went by and confiscated a bottle by slipping it into her cleavage. She made it a joke. He grabbed and grabbed, and she told him he was a naughty boy. They were standing in the doorway, which was such an obvious metaphor. She was out and he was in and maybe he knew he was trapped and maybe he didn't. He tried to keep his desperation tucked in, under some heavy blankets so she wouldn't see. He joked and grabbed, and she stood outside the doorway with the bottle of drugs nestled against her breasts like a baby's head.

Months later, another friend told me he'd gone by John's apartment. He said John had seemed hollowed out. "Like a shell," my friend said. When he drove up, John's bike was there. The shades were drawn and when John opened the door, my friend said it was like something was crawling around under his skin. John talked but his eyes darted, and he moved from room to room like a ghost. John said he was just leaving and pushed my friend out. John didn't leave. I kept thinking he'd get better. I didn't know then what I was just beginning to suspect in my own life. I didn't know the bottles of drugs could empty and empty again and you'd promise yourself you'd stop and then night would come, or day and desperation would stretch its claws and drag you under.

Eventually, John's seventy-year-old mother came out, packed up his things, and brought him back to live with her in Minneapolis. We all hoped this would help. We went on with our lives, sure he'd come back. It was just a matter of time. John was at his mother's house for three months before he dropped down her stairs. It was the middle of the day. She watched him stand backward at the top of the staircase, close his eyes, and lean back like a plank until his body buckled with the impact. He died of a head injury right by the front door.

I sit in front of the computer, staring at the stark words. Grief pulses in me. I wonder if John understood what was happening to him; I wonder if, like a fish, he had no sense he was in water over his head.

IT'S THURSDAY. I'VE been out of pills for three days. I've cried most of the day. Two hours of sleep again last night—maybe three and change. The pills at least give me hope. They give me three or five hours instead of two. They give me something. Yesterday I got groceries and couldn't look the meat counterman in the eye. It was too much. And he wanted to look me in the eye, went out of his way to pause, to hold the wrapped and bagged turkey aloft, to look me in the eye. It was painful to be among so many people, the chaos of energies under fluorescent lights. I kept my eyes down while the cashier rang up my turkey and diapers, the burritos Sean likes. I kept my eyes down while she handed me my change, tried to exchange pleasantries. *Don't look into the garden of my suffering. I can't take it. Please, don't look.*

# PART THREE

*Dr. Amazing*

# "IT'S AN INCREDIBLE DRUG"

*February 2010*

OUTSIDE, THE SIGN SAYS INTEGRATIVE MEDICAL Clinic in bold, black letters. There's a mandala just under the name—an orange-and-red circle with interlocking loops and roulette curves evoking harmony and childhood etchings with a Spirograph. The door is a heavy, reliable wood. No one is outside, and the sidewalk's clean. I step in.

A friend told me about Dr. Amazing. She'd tried for a year and a half to get pregnant and nothing had happened until she'd stepped through this door. Dr. Amazing is an official doctor with official diplomas on his cream-colored walls. He also specializes in endocrine imbalances—hormonal shifts that can render a body infertile or histrionic or sleepless. After six months of work with Dr. Amazing, my friend got pregnant. I've been out of pills for three weeks and have lost five pounds. I'm sleeping two to three hours a night. Nausea is constant. My joints ache. Something's very wrong. I need help. The lack of sleep is eating me alive.

Dr. Amazing's website says the Integrative Medical Clinic uses an evolutionary process incorporating everything from Western medical approaches to herbology to acupuncture. I must be willing, the site says, to uncover the root cause of my "dis-ease." It will take time.

I must be patient and involved. The optimal state for each individual will not likely be another drug or remedy, it says, though Western medicine, with its triumphs and contributions, will not be abandoned. I, as a patient, must not be faint of heart. I must be strong. Dr. Amazing will help alleviate symptomatic branches of my dis-ease while gently moving me toward a shift in consciousness. It will be in this shift that I'll recognize the interconnectedness of all beings. I will move toward wholeness. I will sleep.

Inside, the office is dimly lit. Ikea lamps sit on three tables arranged around a seating area with a dark leather couch and two orange chairs. A large painting hangs on the far wall. It looks like something Van Gogh would have painted as a kid—a rendition of the cosmos; deep blacks and blues in heavy acrylic with red and orange planets and a smattering of stars. A sliding window to my right opens to reveal a room filled with shelves of white and brown bottles. A woman—blond, with hair like spun candy—sits in the tiny room. She's clearly the receptionist and is on the phone with someone who's loud enough for me to hear. She holds one finger up when I enter while rummaging around the desk for something.

"No, no. Truly, not to worry," she tells the person on the phone. "You've got to be patient. If the symptoms persist for more than five days, give us a call back." She makes a lot of understanding noises, little whistles and tsks. She hangs up the phone.

"Are you Melissa?"

"Yes."

"Terrific. Welcome to the Integrative Medical Clinic. This is the paperwork we need you to fill out. It's important to be as detailed as you can so we can get a clear picture of your diet, sleep, lifestyle, and current situation. It's comprehensive, so take your time. Bring it back to me when you're done and we'll get you started."

I take the clipboard to one of the orange chairs. The shadows are so deep, I'm afraid I'll trip on the rug lying neatly in the seating area. Spa lighting, I think. Massage room lighting with gentle waves of music pulsing from unseen speakers. I fill out my comprehensive paperwork. *Sleep?* No, not really. *Diet?* Omnivore with an aversion to places like Olive Garden and the Old Spaghetti Factory. *Lifestyle?* Motherheavy. Mothersunk. Thinking always of the little pills. *Current situation?* I don't know how the hell to answer this. What does this mean? Current horrific situation is I can't sleep and I have two infants and a sometimes husband. Current situation is so desperate I could cry every day for hours and hours. Current situation is my bucking up and getting up bleary-eyed with appendages burning. I feel like the dogs in Chloe's favorite book *Go, Dog. Go!*: "Now it is day. / The sun is up. . . . / Time to get going. / Go, dogs. Go!" I consider writing this on the form but do not. Perhaps Dr. Amazing won't understand. Perhaps he will call Sean and they will take me to some hospital room near the university where the doors lock from the outside. I can imagine this. My own little cuckoo's nest where doctors speak in soft tones and hold my fingers around little white cups filled with more pills.

I hand my paperwork to the receptionist and return to my orange chair. There's no one else in the claustrophobic office. I stare at the outline of the Ikea lamps, the rug reflecting the soot and teal colors in the cosmos picture. It's an ugly attempt at Van Gogh. I look down. I wait. A door opens and a fiftysomething man with tremendous Tony Bennett hair walks out. He turns to shake the hand of the man behind him, who, I assume, is Dr. Amazing. The doctor is smaller than I imagined. A small man with tight khakis and tan skin stretched across his face.

"Thank you," says the fiftysomething man. He runs a hand through his hair. "I hope we can shift things."

"It takes time," says Dr. Amazing, smiling broadly and placing a small hand on the man's shoulder. "But stay the course. We'll get there."

I'm ushered into Dr. Amazing's office, which is shaped like a shoe-box. A broad wooden desk takes up most of the left wall. A small green chair sits next to the desk. He gestures toward the chair and settles himself behind the desk.

"Let's have a look," he says, reaching for my paperwork.

"Oh, of course," I say, awkward. "Um . . . it's just . . . I haven't been able to sleep. Hardly at all. For months and months."

"Um hum," he says, scanning my forms, taking in my lifestyle, diet, and current situation. A very small teak table sits across from me. On top is a statue of the Hindu deity Ganesha, the one with the elephant head. This particular deity is revered as a remover of obstacles and a patron of the arts. It's funny, I think, that so many in the alternative healing arts look to the East for their deities. It would be just as fitting to have some Catholic heavy hitters on the wall. Maybe Saint Catherine of Bologna. She was an art lover. Or Saint John of God. That guy knocks my socks off. But, really, I get it. The Catholics started the whole Cartesian division, the separation of body and mind thing. By having Ganesha, Dr. Amazing aligns himself neatly with those in the East, those who strive toward wholeness and away from the Cartesian mess. It is, I think, slightly clichéd and part of the holistic fashion trend that have people in Ohio saying their yoga oms and buying *It's All Good* and *Namaste* T-shirts in Walmart, but . . .

"So two children?" Dr. Amazing looks down at my paperwork. His right leg—the one farthest away from me—jiggles up and down. His small eyes look up briefly, scanning my face.

"Yes. Chloe's four months and Finch is about twenty months."

He looks back down.

"And the insomnia started just after you became pregnant with your second child?"

"Yes. And it's not the occasional waking-for-a-couple-of-hours insomnia. It's night after night of sleeping one to three hours. I get hallucinations sometimes and my body feels electrocuted. I mean, I think . . . I've never been electrocuted, but . . ." I look over at the Ganesha, sure one of the arms has moved. "Anyway, I've done some research and I think I could have a form of fatal familial insomnia. You know, that disease that's only found in one Italian family somewhere? I've heard that there's a non-inherited mutation variant called sporadic fatal insomnia and—"

"You don't have fatal familial insomnia," he says, his leg keeping a fast, ticking tempo under the desk.

"Well . . ."

"Or sporadic fatal insomnia."

"Yeah, but I read that it occurs primarily after giving birth, and Finch was just seven months old when I got pregnant again."

"How's your anxiety?" he asks. He has brown eyes. Soupy eyes.

"Well, it's fine when I sleep."

"And your son has Down syndrome?"

"Yeah, but that doesn't make me anxious. He's the coolest kid alive."

Dr. Amazing makes some notes. His head begins to keep tempo with his leg. Head and leg are twin bobbins while he scratches away.

"I'm betting we have a cortisol issue," he says. "You're familiar with cortisol?"

"Um . . . stress hormone?"

"Right. It's produced in the adrenals and it's designed as the fight-or-flight hormone. We'll do a test. Pregnancy can often upset the adrenals, and with your pregnancies coming so close together at an advanced age, I'm betting your body just couldn't repair itself."

Relief washes over me. Cortisol. Of course. All those nights staring at that beeping oxygen monitor and feeling constant pulses of terror that my boy wasn't getting enough air.

"What you need now is repair. Your body can't repair itself if you can't sleep, so you get stuck in a fight-or-flight pattern." He scribbles some notes. *So easy*, I think. *So clear. I've been riding high on cortisol and more cortisol. No wonder I can't sleep.*

"I'm writing you a prescription for something called Ativan. It's a strong, fast-acting sedative hypnotic and you can't beat it for sleep. It's an incredible drug."

"I've been taking Ambien and it helped for a while, but now . . . I dunno. I don't like it."

"No. This isn't Ambien. Did you hallucinate or have parasomnia—any kind of erratic behavior?"

"Yes." I give a little jump in my chair. He understands. The Ambien helped for a little while, but I mostly felt half my brain was forced to shut down. I'd wake despite the drug and wander through the night like someone with a brain injury, blurry and disoriented. "I almost drove to southern Utah at three a.m. I was awake, but I wasn't *awake*, you know? It was awful."

"You won't have that with Ativan. Don't worry. You're still nursing?"

"Yes. Definitely."

"Okay, let me check something." He flips through a massive binder on his desk. "Okay, Ativan will be the best. Take it only at night after you've nursed. Ativan exits the body in four hours, so it's safe for nursing mothers."

"*Great*." I feel euphoric. "*Great*. And what about the cortisol?"

"Well, with sleep, your body should begin to regulate itself. We can't get anywhere until you get some sleep. I'll have Babs get you a cortisol test. You'll need to gather saliva in the vials four times a day and then send it to the lab. Can you do that?"

"Sure," I say. "Saliva. Easy."

With this, he flashes a smile of complete understanding. It's a smile of eternal reassurance, one who understands what I've been through—understands as no one else has. It's a smile that has perhaps been practiced and perfected in front of a mirror but is effective nonetheless. It lands on me just as he stands up to hand me my prescription. Ativan for sleep. Broken with sleep deprivation, I do not ask Ganesha what he thinks about this very unholistic prescription. But I am not myself. I am a wounded woman and Dr. Amazing is the one who will heal me. The body will repair and I'll be myself again. *This is a man who knows, I tell myself. He is an MD with a holistic bent and I will follow his orders. We will get to the root cause of my* dis-ease *and all will be well.*

"Thank you," I say to Dr. Amazing as he opens the door. "That was so easy. Thank you so much."

"It may take some time to get your body back to baseline, but don't you worry. Stay the course. We'll get there."

I sleep doped that night and the night after and the night after that. The new Dr. Amazing dope is a buoy and I hang on with everything I have. Sean often leaves early to go skiing and I don't even hear him. I only wake when the door shuts and Chloe startles and grabs for me, hungry.

My girl is becoming beautiful. I've been so scared the little pills have messed with her, my breast a corrosive force screwing with her nervous system, making her a screeching howler monkey. I've worried she'll be an anxious, depressed child, that she'll go Goth in her teenage years, kohling her eyes dark and sliding into drugs and depravity. But we've passed the three-month mark and she's becoming a new child. I can put her down for more than five minutes. I can pee. A tenderness blossoms when I look at her big hazel eyes. Eyes with just a touch of green. She reached for Finch yesterday. She reached and swatted his face and then a smile, big as a rodeo, crossed her face. Beauty. Finally. My girl is here.

# THE LOST YEAR

*2010–2011*

I PUSH A STROLLER WITH TWO towheaded toddlers, a boy and a girl. The boy has lost a shoe and his eyes are slightly crossed. He took the shoe off a mile back and it sits on the sidewalk in front of a house with signs that say *Democracy Is Not for Sale* and *Free Speech Zone*. The shoe is brown and outdoorsy, with Velcro straps and KEEN printed on the side. His father spent forty dollars on the pair at REI. His boy deserves the best. The boy will be walking soon, the father is sure. His boy will walk.

I stop often for wildflowers and hunch over the bar of the double stroller. It lets me rest. I walk a block and then rest. Walk another block and then rest. I can make it a mile this way, sometimes more. It takes hours. I place the flowers between the children. Lilac stems and columbine. Lupine and grand hollyhock. I take time with the flowers, picking them slowly and narrating to Chloe and Finch. Chloe puts her hand out to touch my face. I bend and put my forehead against hers. It's something we've started doing, touching forehead to forehead and rubbing our cheeks together. It's a kind of intimacy I've never known, wordless and primal. And it gives me more time to rest. I can kneel and put my head between my knees. I can sit. I put the flowers in the stroller. I make a bouquet between their legs. Finch squirms and throws the flowers out. I push on, legs dragging like a wounded animal.

I push Finch and Chloe for a mile or more. His eyes are glacier blue, hers like dark honey. I listen for birds. It's spring, after all. I used to love spring.

"Look," I say to them. "That's a sparrow. And that loud one? That's a magpie." Their brains, I know, are being constructed at an impossible rate. Neurons are growing and firing, making thousands of connections a second. And I have responsibility for this architecture. Every sense is registered, and a corresponding tower is being built. Input lilacs and whole cities rise in their brains. Input names and fragrance and touch and a continent emerges where there has been only a vast soup of small, hungry tendrils. Their brains are magnificent creatures. I must help them see beauty and language. I must give them the tools to build a strong world behind their eyes.

Finch and Chloe don't talk, although Chloe has begun making the same chirping noises as Finch. They chirp together and occasionally Finch launches into a diatribe that could be Swahili. I encourage them both. I want my boy to talk. I want my boy to say, "Mama. Papa. Love." I wait for this. Day after day I wait. Day after day I sit while he has speech therapy. And on this day, walking through the neighborhood, I name things. I say, "Tree. House. Dog." I want him to construct me in his world. I want him to own me with his words. Mama. Papa. Love.

I stumble in the street and over small rocks. The stumbling is both literal and metaphorical. The sidewalk buckles in places because of tree roots or neglect. Fingers that long ago dug into wet cement make the sidewalk rough. I trip in these places, trip in others. Blood springs from my knees. I stand and absently swipe at the blood. My eyes grow loose and unfocused. I shake my head. I swipe, gathering more flowers and placing them between the children. "Honeysuckle," I say, trying to gain my footing. "Rose." I hope for cities of fragrant beauty. I stop for the blood and then bend down to grab both of their feet. "Love," I say, squeezing. I stand up and lean against the bar of the stroller. This body is so weak, as if the very air has grown thin around it.

THAT SUMMER, I call several times to get an appointment with Dr. Amazing, but Babs says he's unavailable. I start crying. I'd gone to see him again only two months after our initial visit and he'd increased my dose of Ativan from 2 milligrams each night to 4. He'd told me to stay the course: I'd get better. I've now stuck to Dr. Amazing's protocol for four months, but still my sleep is torn up and I feel panic when night comes. "I'm almost out of refills," I say. "What am I supposed to do?" Babs tsks and hums. She tells me not to worry. Dr. Amazing is on vacation in Costa Rica, but a wonderful nurse practitioner has been taking his clients during his absence. I make an appointment.

At my appointment, the nurse practitioner and I talk for nearly an hour. She's a mother, too—had insomnia issues. She refills my script for 4 milligrams of Ativan nightly despite being uncertain about the dose—"You're sure it's four?"—and when I begin sobbing, she places a soft, warm hand on my back. "It's okay," she says, my shoulders shaking under her fingertips. "It's going to be okay. We all get out of balance sometimes." She gives me only one refill and urges me to return the next month to talk with Dr. Amazing. When I leave, she places a large note in my chart for Dr. Amazing:

*Patient is taking 4 mg Ativan/night. Has run out and needs a new Rx. That (dose) is really high. We need to talk. Something is going on.*

I don't know about the nurse practitioner's note until years later, after I've retrieved my file from Dr. Amazing's office. Like me, it becomes buried. But for now, I have another month of Ativan.

At nights, I look at the pill bottle. It's ugly. A vague evil emanates from the yellow cylinder. The evil seeps out and into the earth under my feet. It crawls up my legs. *No*, I tell myself. *Don't think these things.*

These are the thoughts of someone racked with paranoia. I'm just a dead-tired mother. I must push on. I must get up and go. I tap the pills into my hand. Dr. Amazing promises I'll be fine. Take the pills every night until my adrenals remember what to do. I leave the bathroom and walk into the thin air. I must have patience. *Until then*, I think, *take the pills. Just take them. There's no other choice.*

It's around this time Sean begins running. It's morning and the summer sun hasn't yet made the air hot enough to burn. "I'm going to the track," he says, standing in the middle of the kitchen, his body rigid in black running shorts that fall to his knees. "I'll be back in an hour or so."

I sit at the kitchen table with my coffee. Finch stands, holding on to one of the kitchen counters. He slowly moves his hands to the right before shuffling his legs over. He's a boy on a ledge, a boy building a continent of feet. Sean walks to me and leans over, grabbing my shoulders. He kisses me over and over. These are not the kisses of passion. They're forceful and hard and I feel like he's trying to get an answer to a question he won't or can't ask. I try to pull away to gather my breath, but he kisses harder, pressing his lips against mine, his hands gripping me. Finally he lets go and walks to the bathroom without a word.

Finch clunks to the floor and Chloe crawls over to him. She swats his face and he wraps an arm around her back for the wrestling move he's perfected. He loves the act of pulling her down, of wrestling her to the floor.

"I'll be back soon," Sean says. He walks over and picks up Finch. Finch grabs for Sean's neck and the two nuzzle. "Love you, buddy," Sean says, tucking his nose into Finch's neck. And then it happens. Finch puts his lips together and a sound comes out.

"Pa . . . pa . . . p." Sean looks at me, startled, and then looks at Finch. "Did he just say . . . ?"

"Holy shit. I think he did," I say. "He did! Holy shit!"

"Papa, Finch. Papa! That's right, buddy. I'm your papa!"

"P . . ." Finch says. "Pa . . ."

Sean quiets for a moment, his eyes watering. He hugs Finch tight, then holds him up in the air. "Papa," he says softly. "I'm Papa."

Finch smiles and wiggles to be put down. He doesn't know he's just turned our hearts liquid. Sean looks at me with wet eyes before putting Finch back down. They hold hands for a minute while Finch stands, looking up. *Papa.* He said it.

After a few minutes, Sean retreats to the bedroom. I hear him humming. He comes back into the kitchen.

"Did you move my keys?"

I feed Finch and Chloe avocado and eggs. I take two bites of egg and my stomach contracts into a fist. I push the plate away. In the past month eating has become difficult. I tell myself it's a result of the awful C-section. The resident must have shoved my intestines in wrong, kinking them in some fashion that makes eating painful. I've lost the baby weight and more. I punched a new hole in my belt to hold up my jeans. I'll probably have to buy a new pair soon.

I lean over to Finch, who has moved past his sister and now holds on to the kitchen table, which for all practical purposes is my desk. In the past few months I've pitched stories to *Parenting*, *Hip Mama*, and the *Atlantic* magazine. I haven't heard anything back, but I'm trying. It's exhausting but it connects me to who I used to be. Finch stares, blinking. I lean over. "Mama," I whisper. His hands clutch the metal edge of the table. "Ma . . . ma . . . ma," I say, waiting. He doesn't say it. He said "Papa"; why can't he just tuck those lips in a bit? "Ma . . . ma." I say it again, and again nothing. I feel like an accessory, that lady in the house who does stuff. He can't or *won't* say my name, and this is my failure. I've wiped this kid's butt for two years. I've brought him to innumerable physical and speech therapies and have pureed fruits and vegetables, which I have then frozen into old-fashioned ice cube trays so said fruits and vegetables can be popped out and unfrozen and fed to this ungrateful child. I've walked his sorry ass in carriers and strollers for two years now because he's just figuring out how to be vertical in the world. He'll probably be an ungrateful teenager. He'll roll his eyes and stay in his room, messaging friends about his over-protective mother—a helicopter mama, he'll write. Ungrateful. I can see it already.

He smiles like it's Mardi Gras and plunks down on the floor. I watch him, disconsolate. I'm deep in this landscape of Huggies and nap times, onesies and frozen vegetables. There's no glamour to this life. There's only relentless minutiae and shit or the lack thereof, and no one yet can say my name.

I try calling Ivy but get her answering machine. I call Hollis and my old friend Sedina and then my mother. No one's home. No one's available at the end of the line.

My life is supposed to be more glamorous than this. My life is supposed to be more than the howl of the tired, more than washing-machine-ensconced children. How do the glamorous have children? How do the poets, with their deep-set eyes and beautiful pens, have children? How do the beautiful still feel beauty? "Finch, don't punch Chloe in the head." He looks at Chloe and doesn't understand or pretends not to and then he crawls over and takes her down again.

When Sean gets back from running, his eyes are red and soft. He tucks his head when he comes in and goes straight to the bathroom. He comes out and touches my shoulder with his fingertips. He picks up Chloe and kisses her. He takes Finch into the backyard and walks him through the garden, hand in hand. Later, when we're in bed, he tells me he ran hard at the track, so hard he choked. He went to the high school up the street, the one with a cushioned red track set in a perfectly manicured, fenced-in lawn. He was alone and he ran hard. One lap, two, three. He ran harder. He could taste blood, but he kept running, long legs pounding. Four laps, five, seven. His lungs burned but he didn't care. "Then," he tells me, "I couldn't breathe." He tried to keep running but sobs pounded out of his chest. Finally he just fell onto the grass. "I'm lucky no one was there," he says. "I couldn't stop. I don't know why. I just—"

"Honey," I say, tracing my finger the length of his cheek. "Oh, sweetie." Something has momentarily broken open. Sean leans into me. He's silent for a moment before looking into my eyes. I touch him, fingers tracing his ear, his mouth. He turns and gently moves Chloe to the side of the bed near the wall. He cushions her body with blankets and when he turns to face me, his eyes are bright and hot. His hand runs the length of my stomach. I guide his fingers and then take him in my mouth because I want him. My God, I want him, his body and mine. I take him, and he closes his eyes. I take him, and he grabs my face. He stretches me out to roll on top of me. He's urgent and hard, so hard, nudging my legs open. We kiss and he tucks his face into my neck. He puts himself in me and we fuck breathless and desperate and hungry. I grab his back and try to pull him deeper, try to pull him into me so I won't lose him again, won't feel the great cry of loss that has been our skin and our bodies. I pull him in, and I can feel the sob in his chest, but he doesn't make a sound, just presses his body hard into mine as if he could tear me open, as if he could tear everything to shreds with fucking hard and sad and angry, fucking to tear it open. Fucking to try to make something new.

Afterward, Sean moves Chloe between us. She nuzzles, half-asleep, searching for my breast. I lean over and we're together, and Sean falls asleep with his hand between my legs. We're a circuit—all of us— running together and full of sobs. I fall asleep, my body wrung out with a touch I've longed for, my skin raw and singing like a bell.

MONTHS LATER, SEAN and I decide to move to a new house. Our little shoebox was great as a bachelor pad, but it's beyond crowded for a family of four. Finch doesn't mind sleeping in the hallway that serves as his room downstairs now, but when he gets to be a teenager, he'll need his own room. And I'm sure Chloe will tire of me and won't vote for sleeping in the little nest we made in the closet when she was first home from the hospital. The new house will be a stretch, but we need it. We put all our money in and get a house that, with four bedrooms, feels like a palace. There's a big front yard that's fenced to keep Finch from going too far. The backyard is huge, "big enough to put in our own roller rink," I tell Finch and Chloe. There's a large front room with a wide, south-facing window on the main floor, along with a brightly lit kitchen. Sean's and my bedroom is just off the kitchen, along with a second room that will serve as Sean's office. The kids each have their own bedroom downstairs in the newly finished basement.

In August I'd seen Dr. Amazing for the third and what I didn't realize would be the last time. I told him the pills had worked for a while but, despite the fact I was still taking them nightly as prescribed, they didn't seem to be working the way they did at first. "I'm getting maybe four hours of sleep a night at best," I said. "As a matter of fact, I'm not sure they're working at all." I mentioned that my friend Ivy was worried I might have an eating disorder. We'd met for a glass of wine a week earlier and she put her hand over mine, making note of how thin I'd gotten; like a scarecrow. I laughed awkwardly, telling her I didn't have an eating disorder; I just couldn't eat. I was sure it was the botched C-section. I'd eat and I'd cramp, and it was awful. She nodded, smiling, but I could tell she didn't believe me.

Dr. Amazing talks about the cortisol test I did after my first visit and says it's likely my cortisol is still surging at night. My adrenals are upside down; the cortisol test verified his diagnosis. I need to hang on until they resume their proper function. It's such a relief to have a diagnosis. We've identified the problem and we have a strategy to solve it. I trust Dr. Amazing. My adrenals will stop waking me up at night. I just need to be patient. He mentions the inherent stress in having two infants, one with special needs, *and* losing the job I love. I nod. *Yes, yes, of course. All true.* He gives me the Super Adrenal Stress formula that's chock-full of ashwagandha, rhodiola, and chamomile, all herbs that should help me chill out. He also writes out two prescriptions. Xanax, he tells me, is another fast-acting sedative hypnotic. I can use it on alternating nights with the Ativan. He makes no mention of the note from the nurse practitioner as he hands me enough refills of both Xanax and Ativan to last over a year. He increases my dose of Ativan from 4 milligrams to 6. He writes one line of notes in my chart: *Patient still can't sleep. Six milligrams of Ativan nightly prescribed for insomnia.* I forget to tell him I've begun feeling muddy—my brain unreliable and murky. I forget to say I am losing sense of who I am. But perhaps it's just the toil of motherhood. Fatigue, overwhelm, loss of self and memory—isn't that what happens for a while?

I take the pills and with each passing week I grow more and more invisible until I feel vaporous. I slide into disability. When we move into the new house, the boxes high and solid, I rattle through the rooms, desperate and light as air.

# CAVE-IN

*Summer 2011*

IT'S SUMMER AND I'M RAMBLING INTO the phone. "I can't do it any-more," I sob to my mother. Sean and I have been in the new house for five months and I'm unraveling. I speak in choppy, disjointed sentences.

"I swear, Mom, I can't. I sleep and then I don't. I'll be up for two, sometimes three days and Chloe just had the stomach flu for a week and shit—Sean just wadded up her onesies and threw them into the trash—it was so gross, puke to the rim of the Tupperware and all over me and the couch—and yesterday Finch couldn't say 'puffin' and the speech therapist wrote in her little notebook and it was like he got a D on his report card—a fucking D—and I came home and cried. I just can't do it, Mom . . . I feel like I'm . . ."

"Sweetie . . ." My mom's voice is urgent. I know she will try to find an answer, a clean package that will explain the unexplainable.

"And my stomach hurts all the time, Mom. I'm so skinny. I'm the same weight as when I was twelve. That's fucked-up, isn't it? Who weighs what they weighed when they were twelve?"

"Honey, you're overwhelmed . . ."

"But my muscles and my jaw aches . . . even my skin hurts . . . I can't wear anything but super-baggy sweats and I can barely push the kids one block in the stroller . . . That's not normal, is it? Sometimes it feels like there's a flame all over my body. Even inside my body, like I'm on fire from the inside. It's crazy. And Sean . . . I dunno. Sean . . . I've stopped telling him anything. We hardly talk anymore."

"Honey . . ."

"I've been taking the pills, but I don't know if they work anymore. And I take a lot. The doctor increased my dose two times, but . . . something's really wrong. I just . . ."

"Sweetheart, *stop*." My mom's voice is intense and worried. "You need to call someone. You need help. You have a child with *special needs*." She says this last sentence as if it's the key, the element of overwhelm that explains everything. And I hang on to this. Yes, I think, it *is* harder with Finch. I almost forgot. I love him so much, it doesn't seem to matter but everything takes three times as long and his slow accumulation of language sometimes leaves us exasperated. I need help. It's peak landscape season, so Sean's gone from eight in the morning until five at night, and when he comes home, he's grumpy and exhausted. He eats, plays with Chloe and Finch a bit, and we're done. Most days I'm too exhausted to feel lonely, but I am. Lonely. I'm lonely and so tired and I feel sick *all* the time. Jesus. If only Finch could say "puffin" and understand. If only he didn't sneak out to the street to run ecstatic down the middle of the road. What kid does that? What kid is that fearless? We went to visit the new neighbors next door, the ones from Bosnia, and he walked into their house and flopped on the couch as if he owned the place. By the end of the visit, the grandma was sneaking him bits of chocolate and teaching him how to say "fish" in Bosnian. Wherever we go, people fall in love with him. But he can't tell me when he is hurt. If only he could tell me when he is hurt, things would be so much easier. If only he'd stop running down the middle of the road, I wouldn't be so goddamn exhausted. I start crying again. I look for the bottle of wine Sean brought home last night. I take out a glass. I've limited myself to one glass of wine for most of my life, but now I'm up to two. When did I get up to two? I've got to keep track of that.

"So Christina can't help anymore?"

"No," I say. "She found a full-time nanny job."

"What about her sister? Johana?"

"Josefa," I say. "She decided to go to school full time."

We lapse into silence. My mom is right. I need help. I feel overwhelmed with guilt for not being stronger, but I'm sliding into a hole.

"Call Ann," my mom says suddenly. "She'll help. I know she'll help. She adores you. Call her right now. Do you still have her number?"

And the answer's there. Of course. Ann—beautiful, motherly Ann, whom Mom and I met years ago through a mutual friend. She's closer to my mother's age than mine, but when we all had dinner together, it was Ann and I who couldn't stop talking; Ann, who painted like a master but who struggled with depression and disappeared into herself for months at a time; Ann, who, despite her depression, always felt like summer.

"I have her number," I say. "I'll call."

"Promise me you'll do it now," my mom says. "Please. I don't like hearing you like this. You scare me."

Two hours later Ann and I sit across from each other in the kitchen. Light spills in from the bay window. Finch and Chloe sit in high chairs at the far end of the kitchen table, near the window. They're happy, their little fists grabbing for the animal crackers Ann hands them from the blue bowl set in front of her.

Ann's in her mid-sixties, although she looks closer to fifty. She's big-boned and heavy, with a kind of dark beauty. She reminds me of Elizabeth Taylor and she moves like molasses, her feet gliding over the floor. When we first met, I thought she'd been a dancer. Later, I found out she has fibromyalgia. She moves softly because she has to. She moves through the world like someone who can feel the stillest air sliding over her skin.

And here she is, feeding animal crackers to my children. I marvel at the fact she came. I called, and she said, "Let me put on my shoes," and she came.

I pick up Finch, who's dying to get out of his chair. He wants to walk around the house. He wants to see if he can get one of the doors open to run into the wild. I lock the front and side doors and return to see Ann leaning in toward Chloe with her mouth wide-open. Her eyes flick over and she turns to me with a wide grin. "Watch this," she says. She opens her mouth again and Chloe slowly leans in until her nose inserts itself into Ann's mouth. Chloe leans back and Ann snaps her mouth shut before opening it again with an audible pop. Chloe leans in again and inserts her nose, eyes scanning as if she can get a glimpse of paradise. She looks over at me with a *My God, have you seen this?* look on her face.

"Chloe, what's in there?" I say. "Do you see a unicorn?" And then Chloe leans in toward paradise again and Ann starts making these "Aahhhh" and "Oohhhhh" sounds and Chloe loses her toddler shit. We start laughing and I grab my camera and take a video that we later dub *Chloe's Search for Paradise and the Elusive Mouth Unicorn*. And all this time, Finch is at the front door, pulling on the handle. He's unsure why it will no longer open. It opened before and the world was his. Why doesn't it open now? I explain to Ann that kids with Down syndrome are genetically predisposed to be wanderers.

"It's called 'elopement,'" I say. "If there's an open door, they'll find it. If there's a dangerous street, they'll hunt it down and run right down the middle. And it's often paired with radical nudity. You know, pants in the yard, shirt on the neighbor's fence."

"Is that right?" Ann cranes her head to look for Finch.

"Yup."

"So we've got a three-year-old streaker on our hands?"

I laugh. "And you wouldn't believe how fast that kid can move."

After talking for three hours, Ann and I make plans for her to become a permanent fixture in our household. She doesn't work, and her only son lives in Minnesota—godforsaken Minnesota, where people wrap their bodies in goose down half the year and spend the rest of the year covering their pallid white skin. She lives on a pension from one of her long-dead alcoholic husbands, which means she can paint when she wants and work when and if she wants. And right now, she tells me, adopting my family is what she wants to do. She doesn't have grandchildren, so she'll adopt mine.

I'm teary and euphoric. I'm in love with this woman who makes hours seem like minutes, who can do the impossible right now, which is make me laugh. This is what we've done for three straight hours. We've laughed at the mouth unicorn and then laughed as Finch licked the window, his eyes closed and dreamy. And then I tell Ann about being so desperate for an answer, I imagined I had fatal familial insomnia, and when I bring my computer to the kitchen table to show her the horrific Discovery documentary called *Dying to Sleep*, she doesn't scoff. I tell her the insomnia has gone on for more than two years now. I'm taking my medication, but sleep is still staccato and never enough. She doesn't laugh when I tell her about the persistent smell of ashtrays and the feeling my skin is on fire. She doesn't tell me to try melatonin or valerian or hypnosis.

"My God, Melissa," she says. "I had no idea." And her eyes are so full of compassion, my thin glass heart cracks. I cry quiet, rolling tears for a long time. She moves her chair to sit next to me, putting one hand over mine. I keep crying as she sets up toys for Chloe and Finch in the front room, the room that has a wall of window that looks out onto the street. I cry as she double-checks to make sure the front and side doors are still locked. I cry as she washes the dishes and brings me a cup of peppermint tea.

"The sleeping thing?" I say, looking up at her. "Sean gets angry about it. It feels like he's always angry." I check the time. It's early afternoon, so I know Sean won't be home from work for hours. A quiet desperation builds in me. I've tried so hard to hold everything together, but with this open space of compassion I fall forward in pieces.

"Oh, honey."

"The other day he told me he needed *me* to help *him* put on his oxygen mask. You know what I mean? The whole airplane bit about putting your mask on before assisting someone else? I mean . . . I can't even find my own and . . ."

"He's probably scared," she says, her voice gentle. "It's terrifying when someone you love is sick and you don't know what to do. Try to remember this. He probably has *no idea* what to do."

I stare at the kitchen table and take a long, shuddering breath. Even with the new house, the clean white walls and the backyard big enough to be a golf course, there doesn't seem to be enough space for Sean and me. He's constantly stressed about money, telling me to stop buying lattes or treats for the kids at the zoo, but when I ask how much money we have in savings, his answers grow vague and deflective. "I'm just borrowing from Peter to pay Paul," he tells me. We have our spending account, which he puts money into each month, but I'm blind to anything more than that. And the truth is, I don't have the energy to even think about it. Sean grows more and more distant, staying either in his office or outside, texting at the kitchen table or simply staring off into the distance, rigid and unapproachable. I feel an impenetrable wall building and I'm outside that wall, crushed. Sometimes I try to reach in. Sometimes I retreat, my heart bruised and furious, grabbing at bricks to build a wall of my own.

"Thank you. Oh God, Ann—I think you might be my savior."

"Oh, honey. I can't think of a better way to spend my time than to be with you." She hugs me and glances at Finch and Chloe, who are trying to get past the gate we've put up in front of the gas fireplace. "You *and* your beautiful, unicorn-seeking children."

And we laugh until we double over. We laugh, and Chloe and Finch totter over to see what the hell is happening. There must be a unicorn.

I lean down and tell them we have to say goodbye to Ann, but it's just for now. I stand up and Ann's hug is like manna. She promises to come three days a week for three hours. I feel like I've won the lottery. It's okay if I don't sleep. It's okay if the laundry piles up and we don't get the locks high on the doors right away. Ann will be here, and we'll laugh, and everything will be okay.

Later that night, Sean and I put Finch and Chloe in their cribs. As we walk back upstairs, I touch the small of Sean's back with my fingers. He turns his head, eyes glancing briefly toward mine, and then turns back, continuing up without pause. He gets a glass of water and stands by the sink drinking, his eyes trained to the distance. In the bathroom we brush our teeth, moving around each other in expert silence. I feel frozen and voiceless, pushed away by a force of distance I can't quite understand. What's it like for him to live with my relentless desperation? It must be a kind of terror—terror that has no sides and no bottom and gives him no place to stand. I think about my talk with Ann and wonder if I can be generous when everything in our relationship hurts so much. What can I do with this hurt when it's tearing us apart at the seams?

THE SUMMER DAYS blur. For weeks Ann has been coming for three hours three days a week and on these days I breathe. Ann and I set up the cheap metal chairs in the fenced front yard and leave the sprinkler on and let Finch and Chloe roam. She is a mother and a friend, and I feel I can survive the sleep-slurred days when she's with us. But on the alone days I struggle with feeling like glass. Who knew there would be so much laundry? Who knew one could run out of milk and diaper cream every other day? Who knew the children could find every spot on the hot stove, every crack in the cement, every bottle of Ajax, every unlatched door?

One day I forget to lock the front door and Finch escapes, running down the middle of the street into the wide, glorious open. My God, the freedom and the open sky. His legs running. He's so beautiful with his white hair bobbing, his arms pumping. A teenage boy driving a black SUV turns up the street at high speed and doesn't slow. Terror fills my body as I run after Finch, my screams a wall of sound. The black car screeches to a stop just feet from Finch. The boy's apologetic—he didn't know, didn't see. That night I tell Sean about the incident and it's like he hasn't heard me. "Scary," he says before heading to the office. "Glad you're both okay."

When I get the chance to use the computer, I sign up to go to a conference that will teach me about what makes children with Down syndrome run. The conference is on a long weekend, so Sean says he'll stay home with Chloe. When I tell my mom, she says she wants to come. She wants to understand more about our beautiful boy. One month later, Mom, Finch, and I go to San Antonio and the conference feels like a love-in. The contagion of joy is so profound, I weep openly in the wide hotel hallways. People see Finch and yell out, "He's so beautiful. Look at your boy. Just look at him!" Mom is by my side, laughing and helping me chase Finch through the hallways. She holds my hand in the breakout session that talks about kids running. It's the first time I've felt connected to her in years. My mom is with me; she's by my side. I cry. I have no idea why, but I sob in that room with twenty other parents. We all care so much. At night, counting my pills in the harsh light of the hotel bathroom—5 milligrams, 6—it dawns on me that I'm the one with a disability. Finch is fearless, as full of love and as empty of ego as a monk. I'm the terrified one. I'm the one counting pills and feeling like a failure. I'm the one going blind.

Sean spends the summer running and building walls. People want hardscape, he tells me. They want slate and red-rock walkways. They want to keep things in or out. At the end of the day he sits in his office or lies on the bed and watches *The Walking Dead*, a series about zombies in a postapocalyptic world.

# THE SKY IS FALLING

*September 2011*

I CLEAN THE DINNER DISHES AND drink my second glass of wine. Sean heads to the garage to prep for the next day's landscape projects. I start the bath for the kids, grabbing Finch's favorite toy, an arm-length alligator, and Chloe's teacups. Chloe stays in the bathroom with me and we play, standing on the side of the tub and dipping the teacups in and out of the water. As the tub fills, I walk into the playroom. Wide wood paneling covers all the walls. Before we bought the house, someone painted the downstairs paneling and the ceiling chalk white, so when the TV's on, the room has a Coke machine glow.

I find Finch passed out on one of the neon-orange beanbags Ann gave us. I pick him up and put him in his crib. The kid gets more tired than most, and once he's out, there's no use trying to wake him. I turn out the light and listen to him breathe. Light splashing sounds come from the bathroom. I run in and find that Chloe has poured at least a gallon of water on the floor.

"Chloe," I say, exasperated.

Honey eyes look up at me. She smiles.

"Come on," I say. I pick her up and strip her little body, placing her in the warm water. I'm cold, so I decide to get in the tub with her. I give

147

her the teacups and a large Mr. Potato Head. She pours cup after cup into the head, watching it tilt to the side and sink to the bottom. I'm amazed as it drifts and then drowns. I pick up Mr. Potato Head and dump the water out. I grab the paraben-free soap bought at an astronomical price from the health food store. It smells like oranges. I soap her body and her bald little head. She squirms.

"Mama," she says. "Nononononono." God, she's beautiful even when she's howling.

"Almost done, sweetie." I soap her ears.

"Nononononono." She swats my hand.

I rinse and kiss her head.

"All done, love."

She resumes her teacup experiments. I get out and pull on my clothes before grabbing her favorite frog towel. It's light green terry cloth and has a hood with startled brown eyes that cover her face if I pull it all the way down. I lift Chloe out of the tub and open the drain. Her pajamas are in the bedroom. I wrap her in the frog towel, hold her against my chest, and step into the hall. My foot hits the floor and my legs buckle beneath me, as if they've become water. Chloe's tucked against my chest and I'm falling. Momentum pushes me toward the corner wall. I see it in slow motion—Chloe's head getting closer—the wall a ninety-degree seam that will split the top of her head wide open.

I wrench my body to the right and my shoulder slams into the corner, barely missing Chloe's head. It all happens so fast—two seconds at most. Chloe doesn't even cry, just makes a little squeak as we land and then lie there, waiting to see what will happen next. My body curls like a comma and my shoulder aches where it slammed into the wall. I feel for my legs but there's nothing. Chloe makes muffled sounds. I pull the frog hoodie off her face.

"Honey," I say. "You okay?"

We stare at each other. I lie there wondering if I should yell for Sean. He's still outside, either preparing for the next day's work or having a beer in the yard. I know he won't hear. I keep talking to Chloe, hoping my legs will wake up, hoping there's an easy explanation for suddenly falling like a dead body from a bridge.

It dawns on me I may have a degenerative nerve disease. It would explain everything. I may have early-stage multiple sclerosis. The blurred vision and tingling, the weakness and lack of coordination. All the symptoms are there. I search back through the blur of time: How long has it been going on? When did I go from an athlete to someone on the verge of disability? I argue with myself. Is this normal, falling in this way? Is this the result of so much mama fatigue? It feels impossible to gauge from the inside, and Sean turned his eyes away long ago. Perhaps we've both explained away the symptoms, denying what was right in front of us. It could be worse, I think. A tumor could be growing in my brain. I've heard it starts this way: a simple fall, sensory confusion along with the changes of vision and hearing . . . Oh my God. A brain tumor. That's it. What else could cause such relentless and bizarre symptoms?

After a minute I realize I can feel my legs again. Chloe stares at my face. I bend my legs at the knees and roll up. Everything works. I get up and walk to the changing table, expecting my legs to give out again. I pull out Chloe's fleece pajamas, the ones with dancing monkeys wearing little pink party hats. I bend and re-bend my legs. There's no tingle or weakness, no lingering sensation proving something has happened. I tuck Chloe's chubby arms and legs into the fleece, gather her in my arms, and fold myself into the rocking chair next to her crib. Her eyes close. I rock back and forth, nursing her, feeling my body relax.

In minutes she's asleep. I keep rocking, the muscles in my legs flexing and relaxing. And somewhere in the space of the rocking, a question arises out of the murk. The fall. What if it isn't a brain tumor? What if it isn't multiple sclerosis or a degenerative nerve disease? What if it has something to do with the Ativan? I try to remember what Dr. Amazing told me. They're as addictive as coffee. He knows a man who's been on them for nineteen years and has never had a problem. My body would right itself in time.

But my body hasn't righted itself. It's been a year and a half since my first visit with Dr. Amazing, but my body has gotten far worse. I try to remember if I ever researched the pills. I've always been the researcher, but I was so goddamn desperate. All I wanted was relief. But still . . .

I rock back and feel Chloe's body warm against mine. It's seven o'clock and still light outside. I've taken 5 to 6 milligrams of Ativan nightly for well over a year. And I just fell—my legs sudden pools of jelly over which I had no control. I could have sliced Chloe's or my own head open. But now everything seems fine, like I imagined the whole thing. Outside, Sean gathers tools and sod, gallon containers of penstemon and gold flame spirea. There are loud bangs as he loads the truck.

I put Chloe in her crib and walk upstairs to the office. Sedative hypnotics—that's what Dr. Amazing called them. Safe for the baby. And that's all I'd cared about. Help me sleep and make sure the pills won't hurt Chloe. He assured me my body would repair itself in time: "Until then, take the pills as directed." And I have. Refill after refill, and me like a carp with my mouth wide-open.

I turn on the computer. Goddamn—why didn't I ever look this stuff up? I search benzodiazepines. The computer screen fills with links to various sites.

And my sky begins to fall one chunk at a time.

MedlinePlus is a service of the US National Library of Medicine and the National Institutes of Health. Excellent. This looks good. I learn that Ativan (generic name lorazepam) slows activity in the brain. I don't learn how it accomplishes this, but I do learn that when you hush the brain, everything follows. There's no ability to selectively hush and leave the rest of the body untouched. MedlinePlus says Ativan can be habit-forming. Don't take it for more than four months, they advise. Do take it exactly as prescribed by your physician.

Wikipedia describes Ativan as a high-potency, fast-acting benzodi-azepine. Wyeth Pharmaceuticals brought Ativan to the market in 1977, advertising it as a salve to the panicked, the edgy, and the sleepless. It impairs the formation of new memories, so it's often used in surgeries. When having grand mal seizures in emergency rooms, people are shot up with 2 milligrams of Ativan. Two. I'm taking six. And in paragraph two: "Among benzodiazepines, Ativan has a relatively high physical addiction potential and is recommended for short-term use, up to two to four weeks only." I realize that Wikipedia's pages are open platform, which means they get updated and changed all the time by the Wiki-pedia community. The community usually keeps one another in check, but how much can I depend on them for something like this, something my doctor didn't even seem to know? I reread this last sentence at least ten times, my mind numb.

It's the "only" that gets me. "Only" two weeks—four weeks max. I've been taking Ativan every night for over a year and a half. There's nothing about dosage. I started at 2 milligrams and in the space of six months was up to 6. Doctor's orders. I put my head in my hands. This can't be happening. Maybe it isn't happening. Maybe Dr. Amazing is right and the drugs are fine long-term. I have some unusual symptoms, but I'm also a mother of two toddlers and I've barely slept for what feels like a year. Of course I'm tired. Maybe I'm just paranoid.

I decide to look for another site. I need PubMed. I've known of this site since my brother went to graduate school to study biophysics. In my life before the insomnia and the drugs, I researched everything. Anytime I had a medical question for one of my articles, he'd direct me to their site. As the repository for abstracts on official medical research, PubMed is legitimate and reputable. They're smart and should know a lot about the drugs being dispensed by our nation's doctors. I get the same loose terminology as the first site. Follow your doctor's orders. Use for anxiety and insomnia, and if you feel like killing yourself or taking out your mother or the bank teller, contact your doctor. Oh, and don't use benzodiazepines for a long time. "Long time" isn't specified. Abundant evidence shows prolonged use of therapeutic dosages leads to "true dependence." Who writes this shit? "True dependence"? As opposed to what? False dependence?

I realize I'm using sarcasm to blunt the full force of the information I'm finding. Sarcasm will save me. In sarcasm I'll find the lie and I'll tear it to shreds with my bare hands. I'll laugh in its face. "True dependence" sounds like a hard-core punk rock band. Sonic Youth and True Dependence will tear this medical system apart at the seams. They'll tune their guitars with Big Pharma gift pens. They'll break this shit wide open and I'll throw sarcasm like blood gore onto the stage.

I go back to Google. There's a lot coming out of the UK. I click on benzo.org.uk and in front of me blinks a crushing list of possible withdrawal symptoms. My eyes race down the page and then start again. It's hard to focus. I close my eyes and open them, willing the muscles to work. Everything listed, almost all of it, describes my last year. Even the smell of ashtrays—the bizarre olfactory hallucination I've had since getting put on Ambien—is on the list. It's dizzying the havoc these pills can wreak in the brain and body. Olfactory hallucinations? Who knew *that* was a thing? Ambien acts on *this* brain receptor and you sort of fall asleep. You may also have memory loss and hallucinate the smell of ashtrays. If you take Ativan, which acts on these *other* brain receptors, you'll fall asleep for a while, but you'll just as easily have tremors, loss of balance, loss of muscle control and your sense of self and—oh, yes—you may also smell ashtrays. I close my eyes again. This can't be happening. But it *is* happening. My sky crashes into the crutches I've used to hold it up. From what I've read, my symptoms are caused by my brain's tolerance to Ativan. I've become physically dependent; my brain needs more and more to function within a normal range. Despite my taking 6 milligrams nightly, I have withdrawal symptoms very similar to someone trying to get off heroin.

I have no idea what to do with this information. My eye starts to twitch, something I've passed off as a result of the persistent insomnia. *Insects under the skin, jelly legs, rage, vomiting, memory loss, tremors, seizures, hallucinations—*

*This is too much. There's just no way. No fucking way.*

At the top of the UK site is something called the Ashton Manual. I click on it and a picture of Professor Heather Ashton graces the left side of the page. She's demure, at least seventy, with thick 1970s glasses and hair that looks as if it'd been set by soft pink foam rollers. Professor Heather Ashton graduated from Oxford and has studied psychopharmacology for decades. But her real work, apparently, has been to research and educate about the dangers of benzodiazepines.

According to Professor Ashton, benzodiazepines should only be taken for two to four weeks. Even after one week physical dependence can set in. Dr. Ashton worries about this because in the UK, as in the US, excessive and long-term prescribing happens all the time. And there it is, right in front of me: something called "withdrawal tolerance." With long-term use of benzodiazepines (more than four weeks), Ashton says, tolerance develops. And with tolerance comes withdrawals that mimic the full range of physical and psychological symptoms seen when someone actively attempts to reduce the drug.

*Fuckfuckfuckfuckingfuck.*

The reason I'm so skinny, the reason I battle despair and insomnia, the reason I have a persistent smear of bruises and a memory gone white, is because I've been having active drug withdrawals.

What kind of medicine is this? What kind of medicine makes people this sick? I could perhaps avoid withdrawals by continuing to up my dose. I could become a wisp model, a breatharian who stumbles and falls in the backyard watching the sky until my breath goes slower and slower and then to nothing.

I hear Sean outside. Occasionally a shovel drops to the concrete, making a huge clang. So inconsiderate. So goddamn loud. I consider opening the office window and leaning out to tell him we're screwed, both of us, and could he keep it down? I don't open the window. Rage, aggression, and irritability are withdrawal symptoms. Who knew one medicine could offer so much?

I close my eyes. A huge thud comes from outside. Probably a sack of compost. Another thud. I live with an insensitive monster, a man who shakes trucks to their very foundation without apology. I hate him. I hate this computer. I hate these walls and this vanilla house and this body. I imagine purchasing a pistol at one of the pawnshops on State Street. It would take just a second. One bullet and the Ativan will be blown to bits along with my brain.

And, oh, the blackness of my sarcasm comes in with great heft here. I feel like I should draw up a medical ha ha chart that points to the fact this drug becomes like fishhooks in the brain. There's no escape by just throwing the little fuckers into the toilet. If only I could play out the dramatic scene with me uncapping the yellow bottle and letting the pills slowly rain down while Sean looks on with concern and relief. In my fantasy, he hugs me to his chest. He says, *Wow, that was a close one. Gosh, honey—if we'd only known.* But no. I'm numb. And furious. Based on what I've just learned, if stopped abruptly, the medicine Dr. Amazing has prescribed can kill me. It's on most of the sites in small print. *Whatever you do, don't cold-turkey. Your brain will light up like the Fourth of July. It will be like Fukushima. You'll have a massive seizure and die. If you don't die, at the very least you'll get psychotic. There will be a meltdown. You'll strip naked and people will find you on the roof waving a knife, ranting about the Apocalypse and punk rock. And, by the way, not very many people have a clue how to get you off this stuff. It's a bitch. Sorry. We know you didn't sign up for this. Be safe and good luck out there.*

The Ashton Manual recommends switching over to Valium (the generic of which is diazepam), the original mother's little helper, because it stays in the body longer. There are tapering schedules that extend for months. Or years. Some people experience what Dr. Ashton calls "protracted withdrawal syndrome." And, worse, new symptoms often arise: symptoms people report never having had prior to taking benzos. Crippling anxiety develops and doesn't leave. Agoraphobia materializes where it never existed. Panic attacks appear or worsen. People feel shocks to their brains. They can't remember how to tie their shoes. Some people feel like their very bones are vibrating.

I sit, overwhelmed with the weight gathering over my head. I've been struggling for months and months, the weight pressing in on all sides and me wondering why my chest felt like it was going to explode. And this whole time I'd thought I was just mama tired. All those trips pushing the double stroller up the hill, having to stop to sit on the pavement after three blocks because my legs were shaking—me, the runner, the rock climber, the ox—me swallowed by guilt and getting skinnyskinnyskinny, feeling my ribs and hips sticking out, my ass gone, my cheeks hollow—and the bruises brown and green on my shins and arms and back—all of it explained away because I couldn't imagine, couldn't fucking imagine—

I turn off the computer. It's dusk, and Sean's still outside. He could be next door drinking coffee or talking to the neighbor. I text Ann, asking for her doctor's number. Ann loves her doctor; says she makes house calls and doesn't care about the insurance company's dictates. I'll call for an appointment tomorrow. Maybe her doctor can help me. Someone has to know how to get me off this shit.

I go into the stark white bathroom. We've been here eight months and have talked about painting the bathroom like we've talked about painting the rest of the house. I open the window and look into the backyard. No Sean. I look at the medicine cabinet. The Ativan—those tiny little pills like atom bombs. I can't throw them away. I can't just walk away from this, can't cold-turkey like some heroin junky on a sweat-soaked mattress.

I pull the Ativan out of the cabinet. If I were in a horror movie, it would ooze out of the bottle; it would send me to seizures and crawl across the floor.

The pills are the size of my pinkie nail. I cut one in half and cut one of the halves in half, leaving two tiny wedges. I wash one of the wedges down the sink and put the rest at the back of my throat, swallowing everything with a mouthful of water.

CHLOE'S HOWL RISES up through the house and I shoot off the bed, arms flailing against the dark. In the hall, I struggle for the walls. My little girl . . . something's wrong. At the railing, I stumble and slide down the stairs to her room. It's so black. I don't remember it being so black.

Where's the night-light? The one with little fishes that glow green and blue against the wall. The one with fingers of color.

I skip a step in the dark and lurch forward.

Where is she?

My fingers connect with the railing of her espresso-colored crib. I lean in, stirring for her body. I know her little form so well: the soft loaf of belly, the delicate length of her fingers—like a piano player, I'd said when she was born. I slide my hands under her back and she relaxes into me, quieting at my touch. And then, before I can lift Chloe, a surge of heat burns up my spine. I feel like I'm on a subway platform with a train approaching and walls rumbling with the rush of oncoming air.

My hands slip from beneath her. She rolls back in the bed. Body not my body; legs not my legs. On the floor, my mouth crushes into beige and chocolate fibers, the new carpet tacked down just before we moved in. "Lipstick on a pig," Sean had commented, but we didn't pull it up, didn't change a thing, only put the cribs together and I pressed stencils on the walls—vinyl monkey on a branch, buzzing dragonflies, and cherry blossoms.

Everything in my head is hot and it keeps coming. The room shimmers with a halo of heat and electricity. Colors flash behind my eyes: swirling oranges and greens, hot and pulsing. Something inside flickers on and off. I can't feel my arms or legs. I can't move.

Consciousness shuts like a door. Silence. Then a boom. Heat again, so much heat. The orange erupts, a neon explosion in my head.

Where is Sean? My God, can't he hear her wailing?

A tremor races through my body. I'm alone in this room in the middle of the night with my baby girl sobbing.

Is this what dying feels like? Will Sean find me in the morning, cold to the touch, a milky froth slipping out of my mouth?

The roar rises and fades. Heat runs like a fierce, howling wind up my back. I don't know where my body begins or ends. Colors explode in my vision, raging like a wildfire through my head. The blood orange night turns red and screams through my eyes. The room tilts around me. Consciousness shuts again. Velveteen black. Silence. Time stretches and disappears. A dark figure hovers at the doorway, watching me. I can feel the dark like a cold fabric wafting. I can feel Death wait and then turn. Hssssss. And then there's nothing. A long time of nothing.

The darkness peels away. I lie listening for sound. It's impossible to gauge how much time has passed. Chloe has stopped crying. When did she stop crying? The red and orange and heat are gone. I try moving my arms and it's like dragging them through mud. I reach forward and hoist a leg underneath me before collapsing. Strands of carpet beneath my fingers. Fibers in my mouth. I hoist a leg again, willing my body to move. I slump, carpet scratching my arm, my face. Wait. Raise the arm. Heft the leg. Angle it. Push. There's no ability to formulate a question about what happened. There's no capacity to think of getting help, to think of calling for an ambulance. A part of my brain has turned off. I'm feral, an animal on her belly. I can register only one thing: I must move. After several attempts, I'm on all fours. I begin crawling.

At the foot of the stairs leading to the kitchen, I look up at nothing, not even a shadow. It's so dark. Maybe I've gone blind. I feel for a stair with my hand. I will my knee to move. I'm at the base of a mine shaft, looking up for some promise of light. I lift a hand to the stair, then a knee. Slightly listing now. Crawl up and up.

In the kitchen, my hands stick to the cold tile. Shallow breaths pump my chest. I fall again and lie on the floor, waiting. Minutes pass, maybe hours. Still, nothing but blackness. My hands push again and I'm on all fours. *Slide the hand forward, then the leg. One, two, one, two.* I'm an animal crawling through the darkness. Move.

In the bedroom, I hear Sean snoring. I clutch at the duvet and slump, head on the carpet. After several moments I pull a leg under me before collapsing again. Minutes later I throw my chest onto the bed and breathe in the duvet. Is it the red one? The cotton one with little horizontal ridges? I can feel it in my mouth, the faint lines of fabric. Several more minutes pass and I'm able to haul the rest of my body onto the bed, facedown. After a few minutes I roll over. I can't talk, so I lift my arm and drop it onto Sean's leg.

I can't believe he's still asleep. He can't be asleep.

*Wake up. Please, please wake up.*

Nothing. I wait. Words are queued in some waiting room, unable to travel the distance from my brain to my throat.

Sean's body shifts slightly. He is in dreamland. It feels like he'll be in dreamland forever. I lift my arm again and drop it. The effort is monumental.

I lie on my back, too tired to move or speak. Shadows drift. Everything goes black.


THAT MORNING, WITH Sean rushing for work, checking his cell phone, eyes everywhere at once, I stand. I can walk. In the kitchen, my voice is weak, but I can talk. I tell him about the overwhelming heat and blackness, the colors screaming through my head. "I crawled up from Chloe's bedroom on my hands and knees," I say. "I couldn't talk, couldn't wake you." I reach for the table to steady myself.

"What happened?"

"I don't know what happened."

I'm scared and awkward and I want him to hold me and he doesn't; he stands with his back against the kitchen sink and asks if I want to go to the hospital. My head feels murky. I can't think.

"Do you want to go to the hospital? I'll take you if you really think you need to go." His voice is hard and icy.

Guilt shoots through me. I feel like a burden. "No. I mean, I don't know," I say. "It's over now."

He pins his eyes to the back of my head. He doesn't move, and I shrink away. Maybe I'm overreacting. Maybe it's just something weird with the drugs. My body has become something unpredictable to me. I don't know what's normal anymore.

"I'll take you," he says again, drumming his fingers against the counter, eyes flicking toward the door. "If you really wanna go."

"No," I say. "No. Never mind. It's too late. It's over."

# "KISS THE KIDS,
# I'M SORRY"

SEAN LEAVES FOR WORK. FINCH STARTS hooting. His morning hoots
are the sound of pure joy at being awake and alive. Loud "Whooo
hoooos" filter up, and soon I can hear him laughing. He always greets
the morning this way. I stop in the little alcove at the top of the stairs
and slump against the door leading from the kitchen to the driveway
outside. My heart is a caged bird in my chest. I start crying and once
I start it's hard to stop. I bend over, my body still so weak. I place
one hand on the railing in case I fall. I don't feel like I deserve to
be his mother. He needs someone more patient. He needs someone
who will sing the ABC's with him for as long as it takes. He needs a
mama who isn't cutting slivers off her pills at sunset and praying that
her brain won't explode into fireworks. I cry while I walk down the
stairs. Coffee spills on my leg. Who the fuck cares? It's a small burn.
It'll mend.

Later, I call to make an appointment with Ann's Dr. Kate. They can
get me in at the end of the week. I text Ann that I have an appointment,
but she doesn't text back. She'll be here tomorrow. I'll tell her everything then. She'll keep the kids while I shop for milk and Band-Aids.
Things will be okay.

That night I pull out a notepad to track how much Ativan I'm cutting. Last night's cut of one of the 2-milligram pills into quarters was way too much, I think. I don't want to crawl out of Chloe's room again. I don't want to die. Tonight I'll back it up, shave just a granule so I'll be just a sliver under 6 milligrams. That should work. I chart my dose and put the notepad in the medicine cabinet. The kids are asleep and Sean's in bed watching *The Walking Dead*. And then Ann calls. She's hysterical, tells me she's leaving to catch a plane to Minnesota. Now. The taxi is waiting. Her son has been in a horrible accident—some kind of misunderstanding at a bar. He was drunk, Ann says, but they shouldn't have thrown him into the street like that, shouldn't have crushed his leg. He's in the hospital right this minute having surgery. They'll have to use titanium to hold his leg together. There will be pins and rods to keep the femur in place. There will be screws. He may not be able to walk for months.

She's packed her bags and arranged for someone to watch her dog. She's taking the red-eye and will stay in Minnesota until he can walk. "Goodbye," she says. "Kiss the kids, I'm sorry."

"I understand," I say. "Of course. You must go."

And that's it. I hang up the phone, numb. I wish I were dead. I'd rather be dead than face the night this way. I'd rather be dead than face the rest of the long, hot days of summer and then fall without Ann's laugh to keep me sewn together. It's two months into summer and I've just discovered that the medication I'm on is causing a landslide in my brain and now she's leaving. I have no idea how I'll survive. Why stick around? Why not just walk into some grove and end it? But I can't. I won't. Finch and Chloe are downstairs. I can't imagine leaving them. But more than that, I can't imagine giving in. I want to die, but I also want to kill this thing that has taken over my brain. I think about when I was a rock climber and would climb and fall and climb and fall on a route so many times, my friends would tease me. "Give it up!" they'd shout. "We'll come back tomorrow." I'd hang in midair on the rope and fume. Then I'd gather myself, calculate the route, and try again. I almost always made it to the top.

I walk into the bedroom. Sean's on his back in bed with the computer on his lap. He has earbuds in so the sound doesn't wake the kids. He doesn't look up. I walk out and sit on the couch. I'll watch the day burn into night and I'll shave another dusting off my pills. I'll scour the internet for signs of hope. I'll sleep on the couch when I can and wander the house at midnight and 4:00 a.m. I'll fend off the rage that burns at all hours. I'll see the doctor soon and she'll help. She has to help.

I'VE SHAVED DUSTINGS off the pills for three days. I can't do it again. Yesterday I fell twice in the kitchen while making Chloe and Finch pancakes. And I have bouts of hyperventilating throughout the day, bending over just to try to soothe my breath. In the parking lot of the grocery store I dry heave over the black pavement. Mothers and their children walk by looking and then averting their eyes. I bend over, convulsing, but nothing comes out. Chloe and Finch are locked in their seats. They start crying. Finally, the vise on my stomach releases. I close the door and drive home. I order pizza for Sean and the kids. Maybe tomorrow I can make it into the store.

I decide to go back up to 6 milligrams of Ativan that night. My hands shake when I change the kids' diapers. I'll go back up. I don't care. My appointment with Dr. Kate is in three days. I'll decide what to do then.

DR. KATE'S TALL, thin, and blond, and has a wicked sense of humor. Even better than this is the fact she talks to me without once looking at her watch or giving the slightest hint that she should be somewhere else, solving someone else's problem, curing the world in the five-to-ten-minute increments so often prescribed by insurance companies.

And in the first five minutes I find out she has a brother with Down syndrome.

I've been in her office for over an hour explaining how much I want to get off the Ativan, how long I've been on, how just shaving a few granules has left me barely functional.

"And you're on six milligrams?" she asks again. "Every night?"

"From two to six in the space of about six months."

"And I know you're not doctor shopping because I just looked you up on the Department of Professional Licensing website. You're cleared," she says, smiling. "Just in case you wondered. No red flags."

"Thanks."

"My pleasure. So you mentioned a manual."

"Yeah. So the Ashton Manual was written by a doctor in the UK," I say. "She's done more research on how to get people off benzos than anyone else I've been able to find. Just google the Ashton Manual and you'll find it."

"Okay," she says, typing and staring into the computer screen. "Huh . . . She recommends a complete switch over to Valium."

"Right."

"And you're still nursing . . ."

"Chloe. Yes, I'm still nursing."

"How old is she again?"

"Almost two."

"Okay, you'll have to stop."

"No. Really? Why?"

"The reason for the switch to Valium is to minimize withdrawal symptoms. Valium takes longer to exit the body than the Ativan. It has what's called a longer half-life. Your withdrawal symptoms will be a little easier, but it also means that Chloe will get the Valium through your breast milk." She raises her eyebrows. "So, if you're serious, you're going to have to cut the kid off."

"Okay," I say. "No more drinks at the bar." I smile.

She looks at her computer again.

"I think we can try a step-down process using half Valium and half Ativan. It might be too hard for your system to make a complete switch. How does that sound?"

"Fine," I say. "Good. I mean, if you think it'll work."

"Well," she says, "we'll find out. What I want you to realize is you're going to have to go really slow. I'm not talking weeks or months. This could take two years."

"Two years?" I'm incredulous.

"It's possible," she says. "Honestly, I don't know."

I exhale.

"Just remember: slow and steady wins the race."

"Wow." I run my hand through my hair. It's been falling out. There's a small clump in my hand, which I throw into the trash next to my chair.

"Slow and steady," she says again.

Later that night, Sean and I sit in the backyard. We've pulled the patio chairs close to the house so we can hear Finch or Chloe if one of them wakes. I've asked him to talk and I want to be outside. I want to watch for the tree swallows that come at dusk.

He drinks a beer and stares off to the far end of our property, where his landscape trucks are parked.

"So," he says, his eyes shifting to my face, "how was your appointment?"

"She was great. Really funny. She hadn't heard of the Ashton Manual, so we looked at it together." I wait. Sean says nothing. His eyes shift back to the trucks. "So, um . . . the plan is to switch to half Valium and half Ativan."

Sean shifts in his seat and sighs. "What's that gonna do?"

"Valium is supposed to make the withdrawals more tolerable."

"Huh . . ." Sean looks back at the trucks. Perhaps there's a squirrel eating through the sacks of compost. Perhaps the squirrel's high on the fermentation and doing backflips.

And then there's one of the killer pauses that happens so often in our conversations now. The air between us grows dense. I search the sky for swallows. There's nothing but flat slate light turning the trees into inky sketches against the sky.

"So . . . um . . . I'll start and we'll see how things go."

He hits his knee with the beer bottle. "What the hell is that supposed to mean? Jesus. Don't they know? Why can't you just go to a rehab facility for a while? . . . What about that place near here where all the celebrities go?" He thinks for a minute. "Cirque. The Cirque Lodge. Let's call them. I'm pretty sure Lindsay Lohan detoxed there at least three times. You could hang with the celebrities." He pauses again. "Or let's look around. That one's got to be pricey."

I feel sick. There's nothing I wouldn't give to grit my teeth for a month, to sweat and puke and writhe and then be able to return to my life.

"You know it's not . . . there's no way to do this fast. I've told you . . . the drugs have changed the structure of my brain. . . . It takes—"

"Okay," he says. "Okay. *You've told me.* It's just . . . I was just hoping this new doctor knew of something. . . ."

"She knows about as much as I do. I mean, she knows I can't cold-turkey."

"So what are we looking at? I mean, how long is this going to take?"

"I don't know."

"You don't *know?*"

"Well, it'll take months. It might be longer. She said it could be a few years."

Sean's head snaps toward me. "Years? Are you fucking kidding me?" His eyes are cold, hard, furious—of course. His life has also been hijacked, dismantled, put on hold while I've been sliding deeper and deeper into a hole, pretending not to slip, trying not to slip, with both of us sweeping the shards of our relationship under the rug, because what else is there to do?

"Two years?"

"I don't know," I say. I try not to cry, which is easier than you might think. Benzos have the paradoxical effect of both blunting emotion and offering surging bouts of panic and hopelessness. It's toxic. "I don't want us to have to live this way for long. I mean, it sucks, I know . . ." I trail off, lost. I can barely breathe. I'm hanging on to the shred of our relationship and hoping he'll be able to take up the slack, hoping he'll wrap me in his arms and say we'll get through this together, we'll make it, we'll find a way.

His eyes grow hard as he stares at the horizon.

"I don't want to live this way much longer," he says. It's quiet, this confession. It sounds hollow—quiet and hollow and deadly.

"What?"

"I don't want to live this way for long *either*," he repeats.

Rage and despair churn inside me. A freezing silence descends. I look up: still no birds. Where are they? I frantically search for them in their freedom of sky. Maybe we missed them; maybe they danced their swallow dance one street over.

"I mean," Sean says, hunting for words, "I'm hanging in—I'm not leaving, you know. Fuck. I'm keeping the lights on . . ."

Jesus, I'd thought he'd at least acknowledge how agonizing this is for me—but what was I expecting? That he'd be buoyant? He'd be stoic and loving and unaffected? I feel so alone. All I want is for him to hold me and stroke my hair. But who's going to hold *him*? Who's going to offer Sean consolation while I rage and thrash beneath my burned-out skull?

We sit until the light dims and we become shadows. Sean's beer bottle sits empty on the table. He grabs it and stands up.

"I'm sorry," I say, looking up at him. "I'm doing everything I can."

"I know," he says, pausing, his long fingers tapping the beer bottle. "I know you are." But there's no hope in his voice. If I could paint it, his voice would be a flat black line. He turns away from me and begins to walk to the side door. "I'm going to check on the kids."

I stay for a long time watching the trees go inky and black against the sky. When I finally come in, Sean's watching *The Walking Dead*. *It's time*, I think. *There's no choice. I have to do it.* I put my pill cutter on the counter and pull the Ativan and Valium from the medicine cabinet. I push 30 milligrams of Valium to the back of my throat and swallow them with milk. Dr. Kate and I agreed I'd cut an eighth of my dose of Ativan, so I have to make minuscule wedges with the pill cutter. I squint at the slivered pieces, taking the smallest and flushing it down the toilet. I swallow the rest, choking on the bitter powder that coats the back of my throat. More milk to cut the taste. Siberia, here I come.

# BLAZING GREEN WITH
# NO RED IN SIGHT

*December 2011–March 2012*

THREE MONTHS INTO MY TAPERING DOWN and my ribs have begun to stick out like tiny railroad ties. Dr. Kate tells me my muscles are eating themselves. I have to try harder to get food down. "Anything," she says. "Just eat."

After four months I realize I've lowered my dosage and then raised it back up again five times. Each time I cut my dose, I hold it there for four or five days. Each time I have difficulty breathing. My stomach spasms with cramps; my body snapping shut. Everything feels like it's on fire. I'm disoriented and constantly afraid of falling. Each time, Dr. Kate tells me to go back up. She doesn't know what to do. At my last appointment she confessed she doesn't know how to get me off these things. But how could she? Ativan, like Xanax, is one of the new generation of benzos. It's a heavier, bolder hammer to the nervous system, and more quickly addictive than the earlier generation of benzos.

Both Ativan and Xanax came to market in the late 1970s and early '80s, and both had relatively short clinical trials. What happens to the brain and body after three months or six months of use was for people like me to find out. And as the new generation of benzos gained steam, so did the prescribing. So while Ativan and Xanax aren't *medically* recommended for use beyond two to four weeks, they're *marketed* for treatment of chronic conditions. Prescribing habits followed the marketing push and long-term prescriptions have skyrocketed.

IT'S DIFFICULT TO believe I'm getting nowhere in my attempts to get off the Ativan. Even with Dr. Kate, we can't figure out how to do it without breaking me. I feel made of straw, barely able to keep myself upright. I watch the days of winter pass like landscapes seen through a train window. Things are dark, then light, and sometimes tinged with a rush of green and sometimes the color of wheat.

Sean and I wait for someone who knows something about how to get me off the pills Dr. Amazing said were benign. I call two therapist friends: "Do you know anyone? Anyone at all?" I call countless rehab centers and all of them say they treat benzo detox like other detoxes, with outpatient treatment that focuses on the twelve-step model of addiction to address issues of "cravings" and "triggers" for compulsive use. I tell them I have no cravings, no triggers, only sickness. I'm told to try elsewhere. A smattering of clinics exist in the UK and Australia, but that's it.

Dr. Kate sends emails to colleagues, trying to find someone to help. She calls Florida and California. She calls Washington and Virginia. The answers are the same: *Not my specialty. Go slow.* Beyond that, no one seems to know. Neither of us can believe there isn't more information out there, more doctors who understand what it takes to pull benzos safely from the brain. There are innumerable doctors and clinics specializing in opioid addiction treatment, but this is because the explosion in opioid abuse came with an explosion of overdoses. Part of the horror of opioids is the immense and sudden mortality. Benzos dismantle the brain over time. Instead of a swift and sudden death by overdose, there's a slide into disability. Cause and effect are harder to track because the horror is stealth. Instead of a fire burning your house down, benzos are the thief that steals everything you own a piece at a time.

And the part that's the worst—what Dr. Kate and I have come to understand through our research—is that while the physical withdrawal of opioids is safely done in seven to ten days, benzo withdrawal can be ten times that long. Psychological issues aside, physically withdrawing from benzos can take months. For some it takes years because of the intensity of damage done to the delicate neuroreceptors in the brain. Sean and I have hunted the internet and found no rehab centers with programs lasting longer than a month. Some say they can do a medical swap, transferring you from benzos to Suboxone (an opioid), which would be like setting fire to your bedroom when the kitchen has burned up. This may work for some who have been taking pills to get lit, since Suboxone doesn't get you high, but it doesn't really tackle how to heal the brain.

IT'S BEEN MONTHS since I've been able to read. My eyes can't focus for more than a sentence at a time before the ocular muscles start to shake. But I can see colors and textures. I can see clouds and birds and the wash of sky. Because of this, I start taking pictures of Finch and Chloe with my iPhone. It's a creative outlet, a way for me to play with my beautiful kiddos and a way to train my focus beyond the persistent pain.

With winter has come a furious snow. I walk out the front door and crouch near the window that separates the front room from the porch. Finch and Chloe toddle over inside, wondering why I'm outside, wondering why I'm fogging the window with my breath. I take pictures of them staring wide-eyed and searching through the fog. In one picture, Finch's star eyes look like a picture of the cosmos. In another, the misting of the window allows me to get an image of the tree directly behind me. Chloe's face appears superimposed on a stark network of tree branches. Like a brain, I think, the tree like the gasping arms of dead neurons, splitting and then splitting again against the gray sky. Even in this time of falling, even as my skin burns, I refuse to let go of Beauty. I can't. She's with me, always—showing up in the snow like a bruised lilac on the bushes outside, in the sudden crack of sun through the winter sky.

AFTER OVER A month of hunting for a doctor who really knows how to get me off these drugs, of asking everyone we know, we find someone. I called my friend Janet, a psychiatrist who works at the local veterans hospital. Four days later I left a message with Daniel, a therapist I saw years ago who also happens to be a teacher of Tibetan Buddhism. I studied with him for a while and found his Buddhist training on calm abiding and compassion a perfect complement to his understanding of Western psychology. "Please," I asked. "Do you know anyone who can help me?" They got back to me on the same day and recommended the same doctor. There are two people in Utah who are board-certified addictionologists. They're the only ones who understand the complexity of benzodiazepines. One of them is Dr. James.

Janet texts that Dr. James works as a family practitioner, but he's become inundated with people who want to get off these drugs. There are so many. He's full up, working overtime and then some. She texts that she'll call in a favor. She'll get me in to see him. "Hang in there," she says. "He's the one you want."

Later, Daniel calls. I'm in the kitchen, staring out the window into the front yard. The crocus flowers are peeking out of the soil, a sign spring is coming. It's March, but we've had a sudden warm spell, so I've set up a little splash play mat outside. I watch as Chloe and Finch slap at the water spraying up in a circle. My eyes flick automatically from Finch to the front gate. It's closed. Dr. James has tremendous integrity, Daniel tells me. He can't imagine sending me to anyone else—not with an issue of this magnitude and complexity. Benzodiazepine withdrawal is deeply misunderstood and can't be compared to any other kind of drug withdrawal. Daniel asks if I understand what he's saying, if I understand where I'm headed. Finch starts taking off his swimsuit. In minutes it's over the fence. I try to remember if I slathered him with sunscreen. I need to remember the sunscreen. Shit. I can't have Finch burning his boy parts.

"Melissa?" Daniel's waiting on the line. "Do you understand what I'm telling you?"

I tell him about the past months, about the alienation between Sean and me, about crawling through the kitchen. Daniel sighs and then drops a bomb. I should consider finding friends with whom I can stay for several months. The pressure will be too much for Sean and me, he emphasizes. I need a place of refuge and Sean needs refuge from what I'll be going through. "This will take months," Daniel says. "It could take a year. Find friends who can hold your heart. This is an illness brought on by a medication our culture barely understands. You need to find a place where you can fall apart."

After talking with Daniel, I cry in the bedroom for a few minutes. I'm terrified. Will I have to leave the kids? How can any of this work? I've never felt so alone and there's nothing that can make this better because the medication has been like a stoplight for my neurotransmitters and now I'm tapering off and the light has gone green, blazing green with no red in sight, no red for miles and cars coming in at high speed from everywhere. I feel a burn in my head, a buzzing. *Get yourself together.* I walk out and riffle through the bathroom. I grab the sunscreen.

After Sean gets home, I tell him I need a break. I can't say anything else to him right now. It's incomprehensible. I'm not ready. He takes the kids into the backyard while he works in the garage. I collapse on the bed and a muscle spasm grips my stomach with such intensity, I can't breathe. I fold up, tucking my body against the pain. The digital clock reads 6:12 in bloodred letters. I blink. My eyes twitch. I close them. A searing pain roars into my legs. Pricks in my scalp—the fire ants burning under my skin. This torture—I can't take it. It's too much. *Just bury me*, I think. *I can't do it. I have to. I can't.*


THREE WEEKS LATER, Sean and I make the thirty-minute drive to South Jordan, Utah, to meet Dr. James. I asked Sean to come with me. "At least for the first one. There will probably be a lot of information. Will you write stuff down? I'm afraid I won't remember. I want us both to understand what it's going to take. Please come."

I press the side of my head against the glass window in the passenger's-side door. Gray snow is piled up in small hills on the sides of the highway. I fog the window and trace a happy face on the glass. Through it, I see the chalk-white, empty sky.

I'm forty-two years old. My mother was forty when she disappeared, showing up two days later in the rehab unit at a local hospital. This is the story she retells yearly, on or near her anniversary of sobriety. My version of the story is of moving into my boyfriend's family's garage after finding the tiny envelopes of cocaine and Mom's mirrors with the dusty white sheen. We argued. I begged her to get help. I remember how she got on her knees. I remember her swearing to me the cocaine wasn't hers. It belonged to her boyfriend. She wasn't using. She swore to me. She begged. Later, as she tells it, she drank half a bottle of Scotch, did several lines of cocaine, and drove to the deserted beach near Half Moon Bay. The gun was heavy in her hand. All she'd wanted was the drugs. To crush the loneliness, crush the death inside of her. *Cold metal salvation*, she thought. *Do it.* She was an addict, she told my brother and me. All she could think about were the little packets, the tender cut of the razor blade, the sting going in. She needed help.

And now here I sit, just two years older than my mother was when she confronted her addiction, waiting for a doctor to help me get off drugs. I've always told myself that my narrative isn't her narrative. I don't lie and cheat and abuse. I don't rage against the walls of my life and let that rage burn the skin of my children. I've held myself as better, which is to say I've held myself apart. I spent years studying everything from Carl Jung to Tibetan Buddhism to Vipassana meditation. I wrote poems from the point of view of the addict, the daughter, the mother. I tried each identity, but I could never fully bridge the gulf that had opened during my childhood. I was proud of my mother but ultimately still afraid of her rages. Our relationship was staccato: sometimes on, sometimes off. I loved her even though hurt still lived in my body. I press my hands against my legs. I wonder what it felt like for her, driving to that rehab hospital. I wonder if she felt the shame that I feel now, the sense of somehow failing the people we love the most. I look up to watch as Sean pulls into a large parking lot with a very clean two-story medical complex on the north side. My mom was alone when she checked herself in. I have Sean, but still, I feel so very alone. Sean stops the car and opens his door without looking at me. I'm slow. My whole body hurts. Sean strides toward the building. I walk after him, my steps measured and careful. Neither of us says a word.

Inside the office, Sean and I sit in chairs next to each other. An automatic coffee machine hums in the corner. An older woman leans with her back against the wall, reading *Codependent No More*. Across from us sits a massive television screen playing a Disney movie. There's pink in the movie and possibly a princess. I'm too preoccupied to focus and my eyes hurt if I look at any kind of television or computer screen for too long. All I know is there are no dark mountains. There's no grief and there are no pills.

Forty-five minutes after checking in, Sean and I are taken to a room. The nurse apologizes. Dr. James has been overscheduled. He's moving as fast as he can. My blood pressure and pulse are taken and typed into a computer. Medications and dosages are recorded. I answer the usual litany of questions until the nurse asks why I'm there, at which point I briefly imagine grabbing her by the throat.

The nurse looks at me, waiting. I remind myself she's not the enemy. She didn't push the drugs through the FDA after brief trials. She didn't provide marketing for the drug companies that advertised Xanax and Ativan as a treatment for chronic conditions—insomnia, panic disorder, anxiety when speaking in public or going to a fancy dinner party where you know *nobody*. I take a deep breath, shame an anvil weighing on my heart. "I'm here because I want to get off Ativan." I shuffle my feet. "I've been trying for six months, but I'm not getting anywhere." There it is, like a dead fish. My inability to get off the drug feels like a personal failure. I pull the confession out of my pocket and drop it on the floor.

The nurse doesn't blink. She types.

"And you were taking it for . . . ?" She waits.

"Insomnia," I say, and it seems so innocuous, so easy. I couldn't sleep because of a perfect storm of back-to-back pregnancies with accompanying hormonal storms, despair at losing my beloved job, and overwhelm at becoming a stay-at-home mom. The laundry alone made me weep, the feeling that I had to be a pretty lamb chop, a June Cleaver CEO all bright and shiny as a countertop. I was a terrible, sleep-hung hausfrau, and so they gave me the best sedative-hypnotic around. They gave me the big guns. "You will sleep," Dr. Amazing said. And I believed him.

Sean sits with his hands folded between his legs. I tap a beat into the floor. No pictures decorate the walls. Near the door, a hanging black folder displays flyers discussing diabetes and high blood pressure. We've been here over an hour already. The nurse finishes typing and stands. She tells us Dr. James will be with us shortly. We get a wash of smile at the door before she exits, her blond ponytail swishing behind her.

Ten minutes tick by. Fifteen. I watch the clock. At eighteen minutes, the door opens and a massive man steps inside. He has to be close to seven feet tall, with wild, copper-colored hair. I stand to shake his hand and notice my head is nearly eye level with his crotch. He's wearing sage corduroy pants held up by a belt with an oval-shaped buckle that has some kind of map inlay—blue and green lines intersecting at various points with a red star off to one side.

He flops into the small chair in front of us, long legs stretching nearly to my feet.

"So," he says, flipping through the pages of my chart, eyes scanning every page, "six milligrams of Ativan?" He raises his eyebrows.

"Yeah," I say. "Six." I look down.

He expels his breath and rubs at his hair with a hand the size of Texas.

"So run through the whole thing with me. You were being treated for insomnia?"

"Yeah. Like night after night of maybe an hour of sleep . . ."

He nods and I can see his brain ticking along, evaluating. "Yeah, it can pull you to the brink. Looks like you got to six milligrams pretty quick. There were only six months between your first and last appointments?"

"Yeah. I was at six milligrams by July."

"And he didn't ask you to come back to check in . . . reevaluate?"

"No. Never. He was out of town a lot. He gave me enough refills to last a year."

"Of the Ativan?"

"Ativan and Xanax, but I didn't like the Xanax. He said I could switch it up."

"Wow. Okay. So, let's see, that's six milligrams of Ativan you've been taking for just over a year and a half?"

"Right."

"Every night?"

"Every night."

"Yeah, and it's probably not even helping you sleep much anymore, is it?"

"No," I say. "It sucks."

"Yeah. It's amazing short-term but after that it's a killer. Not much better than a placebo after a few weeks. And you're on a really high dose," he says, rubbing his hand over his forehead again. "But it's doable. I've gotten a guy off who was taking eight. It was rough. Took a long time, but he stuck it out."

I hang suspended on his words. They're like scalpels: clean, bright, and almost too sharp to hold. Fuck. Will I be able to do this? Will I have the strength?

"How long did it take him?" I ask.

"Almost two years," he says. "It was pretty gnarly, but the guy had been a linebacker in college, so . . ." He looks over at Sean, who has a notepad in his lap. "You taking notes?"

Sean nods.

"Good. Okay." He leans back and puts his hands behind his head. "Here's how it's going to go. I've got to ask you a series of questions for my notes and then we'll talk treatment. Cool?"

"Yeah," I say. "Fine."

"Have you heard of the Ashton Manual?"

"Yeah," I say, sitting up. "I read the whole thing online. I actually showed it to my other doctor and we tried a step-down using half Ativan and half Valium."

He shakes his head. "Nope. That won't work. Ativan's half-life is too short. The withdrawals are fucking brutal. And on your high dose . . . no wonder you're not getting anywhere. No, we're going to switch you over entirely to Valium."

"Oh," I say, a half exhale, half sigh.

"Yeah." He nods. "It's gonna be weird. You'll likely have intense dreams and could feel disoriented in the morning, but you'll do fine. We'll switch you over tonight."

I stare at this massive man to whom I'm giving over the health of my brain, maybe my life. I'm terrified, but inexplicably I trust him. Because Valium stays longer in the body, the brain doesn't have as severe a freak-out when the drug is reduced. Instead of the abrupt removal of the emergency brake in the brain, which is what happens with Ativan, Valium edges it off at a slower tempo. I shift my legs against the black plastic chair. Everything in my body hurts. I've tried to get off these things for six months and I've failed. What do I have to lose?

"All at once?" I ask.

"Yup," he says. "You'll be fine. And it'll help." He grabs a clipboard from the counter. "You ready for a bunch of questions?"

"Yeah," I say. I look at Sean, who is staring at the flyers on the wall. "Shoot."

"Okay. Do you have any history of anorexia or bulimia?"

"No."

"Do you smoke?"

"No."

"Do you drink alcohol?"

"Yes."

"How much?"

"A glass of wine or two a night."

"Every night?"

"Pretty much."

"Ever drink more?"

"No. I can't think of the last time I've had more."

He looks at Sean, who nods in assent.

"Okay. Ever use opiates outside of a doctor's prescribing?"

"No. I used Percocet for a few days after my C-sections. That's it."

"Cool." He nods. "Okay, did you ever take Ativan during the day? You know, like if you had kind of a rough day with the kids. Once or twice?"

I'm shocked. I've never even thought about taking more.

"No," I say. "No . . . I mean . . . I just wanted to sleep."

"Yeah, yeah," he says. "Yeah. Of course. Okay . . . ever run short and have to call your doctor for an early refill?"

"No," I say. "Never."

"Okay," he says. "Excellent. We're done with the questions. You wanna ask me anything at this point?" He looks back and forth between Sean and me.

Sean shifts forward in his chair. He clears his throat. "How long do you think this is going to take? I mean, for Melissa to get off these?"

"Good question," Dr. James says. "All right—the best way to do this so Melissa doesn't totally crash and burn is by tapering her dosage by one-tenth every two weeks. She'll taper and then hold. We don't want to go quicker because it takes at least that long for the brain to adjust to the new dosage."

"But what about the places that say they can detox people in a month?" Sean asks. "Melissa called a place that said they could do it in two weeks."

I can't believe Sean is asking these same questions again. I've shown him the Ashton Manual. I've shown Sean PubMed articles and tapering schedules from the Benzo Buddies chat room. He can't seem to digest the reality that this drug withdrawal is different from all others, that I can't just go away and come back fixed. I've done everything I can to help him understand and it hurts that he keeps asking. I want to shrink away. I feel invisible to him, as if my pain is, in his mind, an impossible exaggeration. But then, who could really imagine this scenario? Who could fucking imagine I'd get a prescription from a doctor who assured me it was safe and I'd end up here?

Dr. James gives a snort and shifts in his chair. "Well, you know, that has a lot to do with insurance companies. And some people have to do it that way . . . but I don't recommend it. It's misleading. The brain has a hard time recovering with that kind of quick taper, and the bad withdrawal symptoms still last for months, sometimes years. So, you know, most rehab centers in the US put people on a rapid Librium taper to make sure they don't have a fatal seizure. This is basically wrapping them together with chicken wire and bubble gum and sending them out where they'll get hit with the kind of intense withdrawal symptoms Melissa's having. People think they're all done and they're still barely functional, so they freak out and usually end up reinstating meds or having a stint in the ER. And if you go to the ER, the first thing they do is pump you with more meds. So yeah. I wouldn't recommend that route if you can avoid it."

"Okay," Sean says. "So how long?"

"My guess would be nine to ten months. Maybe longer if Melissa hits a rough patch, which can happen." He turns to me. "You're having withdrawals now, I'm guessing. You know about withdrawal tolerance, right? Efficacy wanes after a number of weeks and then withdrawals can set in even though you're still taking the drug?"

"Yeah. Yeah," I say. "I read that. I have almost all the symptoms Dr. Ashton lists in the manual. You know: insects under the skin, jaw pain, muscle tremors, jelly legs. Everything hurts all the time. My scalp, my eyes, my legs, my stomach. It's like there's broken glass under my skin. It's *lurid*. It's like my body feels *lurid*. That's the word—everything bright and razor-sharp. And I smell ashtrays. All day, all I smell is ashtrays."

I sigh and slump back. Dr. James nods, his lips pursed.

"Yeah. Yeah, I *totally* get it. Okay, so give me the top two. What are the two absolute worst?"

I've never thought about it this way. Everything feels sick. My muscles and joints ache. I'm constantly nauseous. My eyes tick in their sockets. Everything feels off-kilter and stumbling. I take a deep breath.

"It's the insomnia," I say. "That and going into the black. I mean, you know: the times I just feel like the sickness is in every brain cell and it'll never get better and I just want to Glock myself." I rub my temples and steal a glance at Sean. I've never told him I feel this way. Saying it out loud, naming it, feels like the bravest thing I've done in my life. My biggest terror is that I'll lose strength, that I won't make it, that I'll give in to the pain and do myself in. Sean stares straight ahead.

"Okay," Dr. James says. He sits up in his chair and leans toward me, putting his elbows on his knees. "Okay. So listen. We can manage those things. I promise. If you hit a wall of insomnia or you go into the black, come and see me right away. Remind yourself you're going through a *very* intense drug withdrawal. One of the worst. The insomnia and the black are just part of that. You *will* get better. You might fall a little, but we've got stuff in our arsenal to help. We won't let you fall far."

I switch over entirely to 60 milligrams of Valium that night—the equivalent of 6 milligrams of Ativan. My dreams are a carnival all night long—trash and carnivals and blood. The images are fast and furious and bright red. I remember Finch hobbling through a crimson-and-gold circus tent, one leg broken, bone splintered and pushing through his skin, blood gushing everywhere. I chase him, and men's arms pull me back, huge arms crushing me, pushing me down. I'm an animal of pain, mad with my own and Finch's suffering. There's nothing but blood, nothing to stop its flow. And then tents drift by on an ocean, flattened by wind. I'm drifting, and I see Chloe and Sean under the tents. They're drowning, unable to push their mouths past the fabric. I can see them, but I'm tangled and can't make my way over to them. I watch them struggle and sink. I watch them die.

The night goes on for what feels like years, but in the morning I'm able to get up and make coffee without getting sick. I know that the benzos interrupt stages three and four of sleep, but even this is better than not sleeping at all. I'm fragile, and my hands shake as I heat the water, pour the grounds into the press, set out two cups. *How will I handle this?* I wonder. *Because it's just beginning, and no one can save me from it.* I walk downstairs and pull Finch out of his crib. Chloe's still asleep, so I sit on the couch with Finch—my beautiful boy—in my arms. He's warm, snuggling into the crook of my arm, tracing the line of my finger.

I ask myself why I choose to stay alive. I can't even feel the *me* that was before all this—the artist, the explorer, the mother. I'm an evaporating woman; I'm turning to mist. Finch's finger touches mine and the burn in my brain flares up. I have the feeling that I'll never be the same again. All I know is that I must make it through. I know that after a night of terror or a day of being broken by pain, I will get up. I always get up. This is the choice I've made. There's no way for me to control the suffering. It will come and come, like inevitable waves on a furious shore. The only thing I know is I can do things to keep the pain from breaking me. I look into Finch's sleepy eyes, the way his gaze holds me like a Zen master. He reaches out and touches my breastbone. "Mama," he says, his blue eyes locking on mine. Grief and love sear my heart. This boy. I trace the line of his delicate nose, the blond hairs of his eyebrows. Rather than stand in horror at the shore of my own suffering, I know that I must keep my eye trained on the beautiful. Somehow, in each moment, or the moment after, I have to look beyond myself. I curl my fingers around Finch's and watch the play of light around our hands until golden sunlight fills the room.

# SIBERIA

*March–April 2012*

AFTER TALKING WITH THE TIBETAN LAMA–THERAPIST Daniel several weeks ago, I asked Sean to come with me so Daniel could explain everything to him that he'd explained to me. We meet Daniel in his office just days after our appointment with Dr. James. The whole idea of my living somewhere else during the detox felt like such a radical move I needed Sean to hear it from him. Daniel repeats to Sean what he'd said to me. There are no rehab centers in the US equipped to deal with the kind of withdrawal I'll go through. We'll have to create our own. I'll need, Daniel tells him as he told me, a place where I can be alone with my agony, able to focus on surviving. No one can do it for me. No one can take the burn from my skin, the nausea, the constant feeling something is vibrating inside my body. I'll rage when the sickness hits and Sean will need respite from what I'm going through. Do we know anyone? We'll need to put the kids in day care. We'll need someone to help us with the most basic of things: laundry, shopping for diapers and milk, keeping order when our world feels shattered. Sean's mother, Sharon, will come. He can barely stand it, but she will come. She wants to help.

After our conversation with Daniel, Sean and I decide it's best that I detox at Hollis and Jerome's house. I considered a few friends, but Hollis and Jerome are the only friends I know who don't mind my brain is on fire. Hollis has the protective mama love I need. And the fact that Jerome is a psychiatrist means there will be someone around who can step in if there's a major medical or psychiatric issue. I don't expect psychosis, because I'm going very slow, but benzos are unpredictable, and the brain can scream when you pull them out. I hope I won't need Jerome's expertise, but knowing he's there if I go off the rails means everything.

The room Hollis and Jerome have decided to give me in their house used to be their daughter's room. I find daughter memorabilia everywhere: Inuit dolls and stuffed bears, sharpened pencils in the desk, a small gold trophy celebrating her 4.0 GPA from eighth grade. I'll sleep in the antique sleigh bed and the butter- and lilac-colored walls will soothe me. The room is just off the hallway that leads to a guest bedroom and then to Hollis and Jerome's bedroom. It'll be private but close to them in case I need help. The bed faces a big window that looks out onto a tiny crumbling basketball court set in front of a thick wall of Gambel oak bushes and aspen trees. Vines have curled their way around the window, giving homes to any number of bird families, who chirp throughout the morning. I have a closet next to the bookcase and smaller windows near the ceiling on the wall opposite the bookcase. The room feels illuminated with light and birdsong. I have space to hurt here. I can be held by these things.

I bring three boxes of clothes and books that friends have recommended to keep me buoyant. A friend gives me a small statue of a white wolf with her babies. She says I'll need to be fierce. I'll need to meditate on the wolf. I've placed Pema Chödrön's *The Places That Scare You* on the little bookcase on the east wall. Next to it is a book about sitting with people in hospice. I have a book of poetry by E. E. Cummings. This will be a time lacking punctuation. It will be a time to thank God every day, because if I don't, I will forget how God feels. I must remember this. I have pictures of Chloe and Finch and an empty journal I've titled *Siberia*. I have the stuffed purple-and-white unicorn Ann bought me at Toys "R" Us. She feels guilt for being gone for over seven months, but her son has recovered and has a solidly rebuilt knee. I tell her that having her back is enough. The unicorn is enough.

I'll plan to get up at 5:30 a.m. and drive to my house before Chloe and Finch wake. We've found a Presbyterian day care down the street that will take both Finch and Chloe. They will stay, painting and playing tag, while I detox in the butter and lilac room. But in the mornings and evenings I will be with them. Sharon will play blocks with Finch and do the dishes. Hollis and Jerome will give me a refuge, they say, for as long as is needed. Love will abound.

Sean and I will do this. Against all odds, we'll make it. Years from now, people will marvel at our tenacity. They'll ask how we survived the kind of thing that can shackle and ruin, that can rend a family at its core. We'll be quiet and grateful; we'll know how many like us are still struggling—how many are in the trenches, scrabbling, looking blindly for some promise of light. *We're so lucky*, we'll think. *We've taken the severed threads of illness and destruction and stitched them into a new story. Can you see us inside this story? Can you see us holding our children high, the bright spring sun glittering in our hair?*

SHARON ARRIVES AT four o'clock in the afternoon the day after I move in with Hollis and Jerome. We shop for supplies—toilet paper, milk, eggs, burritos, boxes of wipes. She helps me stack the dry goods in a storage closet downstairs at my house. Sharon will work until her fingers split. She's like a river, running all the time. Helping us gives her direction. She flows forward, stacking diapers and wipes, cleaning counters and folding endless loads of laundry. We're preparing. It's all we know to do. Cook and freeze, stack and wipe. Chloe and Finch start day care next week. They'll color and sing songs about the alphabet, and I'll clutch at my body in the daughter's room. Sean will go to work, and Sharon will wash the dishes and play solitaire on her iPad until we arrive home. We'll have snack packs and diapers and we'll close our eyes and wait like a family stuck inside a car that's stalled on some train tracks. There's a whistle in the distance. The train is coming.

IVY GOT ONLINE and looked to see if there was anyone who had published a book about getting off any kind of prescription drugs. Our friendship after the *Wasatch Journal* closed became strained with the insomnia and the sickness. She hasn't known what to do, she tells me over the phone. I begin actively detoxing in a week and she says she's felt scared and unsure of how to support me. Looking for someone who's been through something similar is her way of trying to help. So she hunted for stories and they were there: horror stories; stories of loss and being trapped like a monkey in a medical laboratory. But Ivy kept looking and discovered a book that was on the verge of hitting bookshelves by a man who was a world-class rock climber. It's called *Death Grip: A Climber's Descent from Benzo Madness*. Ivy tells me to search for him. Even though the book isn't out yet, I can find him. There are ways.

And so I search for Matt Samet on LinkedIn, "the world's largest professional network" and finder of obscure writers. And there he is, like a goddamn sunrise—someone who's been there and made it out. Someone who knows. I need to contact this Matt Samet, killer climber and writer. I need him because he is part of the horizon I'm looking toward. He writes me back after the first email. I'm ecstatic. He's a light in a darkness that felt it had no end.

I write Matt several times a week. He tells me about the occasional people who contact him, supposedly seeking advice for benzo withdrawal who, upon investigation, he discovers are employees in the pharmaceutical industry. He warns me to be cautious. The woman who helped him understand how to withdraw from benzodiazepines was entrapped by someone just like this. He tells me that they asked for her help and she sent them a link to the Ashton Manual. Despite the fact they'd misrepresented who they were, she was brought to court for dispensing medical advice. She ended up winning but the court case took years and her practice as a therapist was destroyed. "You can be supportive," Matt says. "But be careful." I devour his messages. He's the first person I've met who understands the kind of dark I'm in. He tells me I can write or call anytime. "It's the kind of horror that's impossible to imagine," he says in his email. "But if you've been in withdrawal tolerance, you've probably seen how bad it can get. It's just going to take a lot of time."

I tell him that Finch is three and a half and Chloe just two. I tell him of the morning just days ago when Finch spoke his first full sentence. I was playing with him in his crib and had left for a moment to pick up his Hug Me puppy. "Mama," he yelled. "Where are you?" I picked him up and sobbed. Chloe wandered in wondering what all the fuss was about and I tickled her and cried harder. Matt writes, "My heart goes out to you having to do this with two toddlers. We have a little one too, six months old. You're giving your kids a chemical-free mother back, which is an amazing gift indeed."

Sean has asked me to wait until May to start detoxing. He needs to get prepared, he tells me. He wants to be ready for his landscape season and he needs time. Our conversations about what is coming are dry and practical: "Who will pick up the kids?" "Who will make dinner?" "How long will it take until this is over?" I realize I've stopped telling him anything beyond the logistical and he long ago stopped asking. I don't tell him when the fire consumes my skin. I don't tell him of the beautiful songs Chloe sings in the bath. We're enduring. I tell him he'll need emotional support, a therapist, something. "It's so much," I say, reaching. But even this gesture falls like a leaf against a stone wall.

"Yes," he says, looking past me. "I don't know . . . maybe. I'm just trying to make it through each day."

PART FOUR

*Great Balls of Fire*

# DOWN BY FIVE

*May 2, 2012*

MY OFFICIAL TAPERING UNDER DR. JAMES'S supervision has started. I dropped five milligrams of Valium last night, which is close to 10 percent of my dose. There should be a poem here, something to commemorate getting back the brain. But who am I kidding? I've lost my own words, but the poets still hold me. Today I remembered a quote by the Chilean poet Pablo Neruda: "In the house of poetry nothing endures that is not written with blood to be heard with blood."

Dr. James says I'll probably feel like shit in a few days, once my brain has registered the missing tenth of a milligram; then I'll have four to five days of being sick and on fire. After that, I should start to slowly regulate before preparing to drop again. It will go on like this for the next ten months, possibly longer. It's impossible to get my head around this, so I don't try. Trying to comprehend is simply inviting the mind to torture.

On day two, Sharon and I take the kids to the zoo. Finch is wild, throwing his little body down the wide walks and yelling for the elephants. My diaphragm jackknifes a few times—once near the rhinos and once on the carousel. I hold Chloe on her carousel giraffe. I touch her soft skin, trying to drink it in with my fingertips. My breathing stalls for a moment as my diaphragm seizes, hard as a rock. I look at Chloe—those full lips, that open laughter. After a few moments, my breathing shudders back to life.

After dinner Sean and I sit alone in the backyard. I feel so lost around him now. He asks me how I'm feeling, and his asking feels flat, his tone neither rising nor falling, his eyes pinned open.

"I can feel it coming," I say. "The ants under the skin, you know. And I'm sick to my stomach, but it's not too bad. I ate some grapes this afternoon."

Silence. The wall between us has texture now. I can feel it.

"Well, if it makes you feel any better," he responds, "I've had a migraine all day."

On the last night of the first week, I am up and down for hours. Just after midnight, a searing pain. The right side of my neck is in a steel trap. I can't lift an arm. I can't move. Breaths pump my lungs like a bird's wings, frantic for air. Delirium of pain. I blink at the walls. I know these walls. I'm in the daughter's bedroom at Hollis and Jerome's house. The walls here are safe. It's night. I'm here because . . . *fuck, it hurts . . .*

*This is the drugs. You'll be okay. It's just a muscle seizure. The emergency brake has been released and the brain's going haywire, everything's haywire and just hangonhangonhangon . . .*

I lie in the dark. Finally, I can lift my right arm up to squeeze the side of my neck. Send signals to the brain to relax. A thread of pain shoots up to my eye. *Squeeze hard.* After thirty minutes, I can move my head a bit. Sleep comes. By the time my alarm rings to get me up, the steel trap in my neck has let go.

I climb out of bed and pull my mama pants on, the ones that don't hurt my hypersensitive skin. I can't stand anything tight or scratchy. I'd wrap myself in clouds if I could. At 6:00 a.m. I'm out the door. Hollis and Jerome's house is tucked against the foothills at the eastern edge of Salt Lake City. My drive home takes me closer to the center of downtown but it's no more than ten minutes, so I can get back before the kids wake.

At 9:00 a.m. I put Finch and Chloe in their car seats and drive to the airport. I tell them Grammy is flying here on a big plane and that she'll stay through the weekend. My mom wants to help, her heart open and bleeding at what I'm going through. She understands. She has raged and fought and lied but she will be here to hold my children. If I can bear it, my mother will hold me. There are no words to capture the gratitude I feel that I can break in front of her. I'm a great, stumbling wash of humility. *Mama—she's here to help.*

She's in the air over our heads, I tell Finch and Chloe. She's waving. Sean is doing errands and Sharon is downstairs at my house folding little pants and dresses, socks smaller than the palm of my hand.

At the airport, Mom stands at the curb with her dogs, Olivia and Zack. I help lift her luggage into the back of my car and she slides into the passenger seat. The dogs are a flurry in her lap. They scratch the window. She twists her body around to see Chloe and Finch. They both grin and stare at her. She tickles their feet and turns back to me.

"How *are* you?" she asks.

And this question is the thing that's most difficult. Friends have asked the same thing and I pause, falling into a sinkhole of doubt. Do I tell them? Do I try to describe what it's like? My mother looks at me, concern dark in her face. I begin telling her about last night—the muscle seizure, the feeling I won't make it out—but her dogs can't settle. They try to get into my lap, then try jumping into the back seat. They're everywhere, little dog nails digging into my leg. My mother admonishes them, caught up in their flurry. I drive.

At home, Sean stands in the kitchen surveying the groceries he's bought. He wants to cook tonight. My mother is here and it's spring and he's going to grill steaks and make a Caesar salad. Sharon squeals when she sees my mother and the dogs. Her voice gets high and she peppers my mother with questions. My head pounds. What time is it?

Four thirty p.m.? I have four more hours until the kids are in bed and I can retreat to my new home. Four hours. I take my mother's luggage into the guest room and stand there. An electric shock pierces my right eye and shoots across the top of my head. After a minute it fades. I search the room. Pillows—goddamn, we need pillows. My mother has a bad back. I mumble this as I walk through the kitchen, skirting around the whirlpool of conversation that Sharon and my mother have become. It's cool and dark downstairs. Sharon's blankets are heaped on the couch. I'll just sit for a minute. My head pounds. Heartbeats throttle my chest. I know this feeling. It will get better. *Just wait. Take deep breaths.* I hear footsteps over my head. Cabinets slam. Why does Sean always have to make so much goddamn noise? My stomach churns. *No, no, no. Don't throw up.* I close my eyes and put my palm against my forehead, squeezing as hard as I can.

"Honey?"

It's my mom. She's standing in front of me, her eyes wide with worry.

"Sweetie, are you okay?"

I lose it. Everything—the frenetic whirl of conversation, the piercing slam of drawers and cabinets, the barking of the dogs—

"I'm here," Mom says, sitting next to me and holding my hand, which is now clutching hers. "I'm here, honey. Go ahead and cry." And I do, sobs rushing out of the small crack I've given myself to fall apart. I shove my fists into my eyes and try to be quiet. All this sobbing—I don't want Chloe and Finch to be scared. And Sean— fuck, Sean—he's sick of it all, he can't stand it, he's vacant and gone and, jesusfuck, I'm losing it—

My mom holds my hand in both of hers while I cry. Her hands look like mine: small, tapered fingers; veins like little blue branches. I tell her I don't know if I can take it. I don't know how—

My breath catches in my throat. I feel separated from my body— not in, not out, but drifting somewhere between.

Mom scoots closer. Her body warms me. Just having her hand, her leg next to me, helps. I close my eyes and breathe evenly.

"Do you want something to drink?"

It's Sean. He's standing rigid next to the couch. They both want to help and none of us knows what to do.

"Yes," I say. "That would be nice. Thank you."

Minutes later he's back down with a cup of mint tea and a thin slice of sourdough bread. I'm crushed and buoyed. Sean goes back upstairs and I sip the tea. Mom stays with me, holding my hands. She rubs my neck.

"You will get through this," she tells me. "It will be hard, but I'm here and Sean is here, and we love you, and you *will* get through this." She promises she'll come one weekend a month—more if she can afford it.

I nod, hanging on to her words. I've never truly understood what it was like for my mom to stand at the edge of an ocean, wanting to end it all. I knew that she wanted to, knew that she's tried, but it was always this horrific abstraction to me. When I was seventeen, I remember waking one morning to discover my mom had mangled one of her wrists with a knife. There was a gauze bandage covering it. Her face was ghostly. I didn't understand then, but I understand now. There have been times I've felt the pain might be too much for me, times I've wondered if it would be easier for everyone if I just ended it. I understand now that despair dragged my mother under. And despair, coupled with the unmooring force of drugs, held her down until there was nothing left. I hold tight to my mother's hands. I can feel a lessening of what stands between us. My mother's hands are soft, and she holds me with my pain, and we are together because I am allowing it. *This is how it is now*, I think. *I'm transparent. There's nowhere left to hide.*

I'VE DROPPED TWICE now—down to 48 milligrams of Valium from 60. Dr. James said exercise will be the only way to get good chemicals into my brain. I will erupt into a rage of fire without them. And it's true. There were two days last week when I didn't push my stick legs and joints up the hill and on those days my muscles seized into knots. My nose bled for hours and I wanted to punch someone, anyone, hard in the face.

I can feel the withdrawals coming when there's a burn under my skin, as if multiple layers of bees are trapped in the dermis and furiously trying to get out. This is the first sign I'm in trouble. When the bees gain in intensity, the benzo dogs in my brain come out. The benzo dogs are like abused fighting dogs taught to rip each other to shreds, devoid of anything but fury. When the benzo dogs come out in me, the only thing I can do is walk, hard and fast. Best not to talk, best not to interact. I walk every day, even if it's at a slant, even if my muscles still seize up. I tell Matt that I only feel a semblance of normal after I've exhausted my body. Otherwise, it's surges of fury or despair. I tell him of the time Sean and I argued and I ran outside to take a two-by-four to the cinder block garage. This was my worst fit of rage, before I even started to taper down. I was in acute withdrawal tolerance—swallowing 6 milligrams of Ativan but experiencing full-fledged withdrawals. I didn't understand what was happening to me and had never felt such explosive rage. I tell Matt how much I feel like a wild animal, alternately cowering and flashing my teeth. I'm apologetic, but Matt writes back immediately, "I know what you're talking about with the rage thing: an eruptive boil, a simmering madness, dissociated and wrathful." He tells me to hang on. This is the pattern. You drop your dose; you rage and boil and weep. Then you stabilize and two weeks later you drop again.

I'VE BEEN THE literary arts coordinator for the annual Utah Arts Festival for over a decade. The festival isn't until late June, and the job lasts only a few months, but Sean thinks I should drop it. I tell him I can't. It's a thread of my old self that makes me feel like maybe, just maybe,

I'll find that person again. So when the executive director calls and asks if I'll do poetry in the video they're putting together to promote the festival, I reply with an unequivocal yes. I will sleep and walk hard so I don't shiver. I will hold myself upright so I can be that person again—if only for the night.

I leave Sean, Sharon, and the kids on Saturday and go downtown to meet Lost Childe Productions, a gentlemanly and hilarious crew of videographers. We take the elevator to the sixteenth floor of Salt Lake's Walker Center, one of the highest buildings in downtown. We're asked to sign long waivers before being allowed to go to the top of the building. The building is topped by a sixty-four-foot weather tower that flashes blue or red to indicate clear skies, clouds, rain, or snow. We're there at sunset. A jazz ensemble plays at the Gallavan Center, just blocks away, giving us what feels like a personal concert as we stand looking out over the city.

I wear my plum-colored dress and quasi–combat boots and shout my poem into the night. The videographers have set up a ladder for me with a box to stand on to get me as high as possible. They position themselves just a few feet below me, cameras pointed up to catch the bright neon of the sign rising up. It's sunset, the time I usually wind down to sleep, but I've planned for the day. I've been able to exercise and then sleep for hours because Sharon watched the kids for the afternoon. I'm able to reclaim my poet heart for at least one night, I realize, because of the mother love of Sharon, my mom, and Hollis, who opened her home to me.

When it gets late and the nausea and shivering start, I think, *Just hold on to the handrails . . . you can sleep tomorrow, and you will be better.* I realize that tonight I don't feel mama lost. I stand on top of the wood box they've brought to lift me into the neon red and blue, and I feel gifted to have so much love in my life. My emotions have been hyper-inflamed, pyrotechnic, and ugly, but tonight I'm brought to my knees with love. It's shocking to feel this set against a body that burns. When I get back to the lilac butter room, my nose doesn't bleed. There are no pit bull jaws in my stomach, and I fall asleep easily for the first time in months.

I'VE BEEN DETOXING for six weeks. Sean, Sharon, and I have gotten into a rhythm. We are an unstable trio, but we're surviving. Sean spends his days planting sod and trees and coming home to play with the kids before losing himself in the garage. Sharon sleeps and cleans and runs errands when I can't do them. I make the meals, take the kids to day care, and work the detox. It's become my job, my only focus—that and making sure Finch and Chloe have no idea I'm sick. This is my ultimate goal, beyond the withdrawal: to make sure there is as little disturbance to the kids as possible.

And then one morning, after waking at six and driving to the house, I arrive after Chloe has woken. It's 6:30 a.m. As I pull her from her crib, she asks, "Mama, where do you go at night?" A cold current runs through my body. I sit in the rocking chair and hold her on my lap. My honey girl; my girl who knows.

"I go to Hollis and Jerome's house," I say. And I wait. I know I have to be honest and I know I can't tell her the truth.

"Why?"

"Sweetie . . ." I pause. I stroke her blond head. She has very little hair still at two and a half, but one long strand has grown down her back several inches long. I twine it between my fingers. "I'm just a little sick. My doctor says I need lots of sleep and . . . when I sleep at Hollis and Jerome's house, I sleep well."

"Can't you sleep here?"

"I can, but right now I sleep so wonderfully at their house that Daddy and I decided I'll spend the nights there for now. It will help me get better."

"Oh," she says, eyes sleepy. Her fingers touch the hollow space on my neck, the little dip between my collarbones. "But you'll always come back?"

"Yes, honey," I say. "I'll *always* come back. I promise you that."

"Okay," she says. And that's it.

Later that week, Hollis tells me they'll be having dinner guests. She and Jerome have been supporting a local environmental group. There's a big fundraiser on Friday and the coordinators will be coming over for dinner. Peter Yarrow of the group Peter, Paul and Mary will be here.

"You're welcome to join us for as long as you like," Hollis says. "I'm making my chicken paprikash."

"I'd love to," I say, smiling. Hollis and Jerome love to entertain and they always include me, knowing that I'll stay and enjoy the warm conversation of the evening until I can't.

That Friday, after putting Finch and Chloe to bed, Sharon and I stand in the kitchen talking about her sinuses. She often has problems with her sinuses and worries it could mean something significant about her immune system. She's either clogged or runny and it worries her. It could be indicative of a larger problem. This kind of conversation drives Sean crazy. He can't stand her running stream of health complaints, but it doesn't bother me. I understand this is her vehicle for anxiety, and she drives it until someone tells her it will be okay. I tell her I don't think she has to worry. Pollen counts are high. I'll get her allergy medication in the morning when I stop by the grocery store. She seems relieved. I tell her Sean will be taking two nights off a week, starting tomorrow night. He's told me he needs to get away and I've agreed because I know it's true.

Outside, Sean stands in the dim summer twilight staring into his truck. He's too far away to hear me yell, so I wave and wait. When he doesn't see me, I simply turn around and get in my car. Our goodbyes have become perfunctory gestures. We wave and nod and turn away from each other.

The drive to Jerome and Hollis's house takes ten minutes. Six people sit around the dinner table. The fundraiser was successful. A huge platter of chicken paprikash sits in the middle of the table and plates are heaped with warm bread and salads. Someone has asked Peter Yarrow about the song "Puff the Magic Dragon." They want to know once and for all if the urban lore is true. Was it a drug song? Was it marijuana disguised? "Jackie Paper," someone says with emphasis, bringing pinched fingers to mouth as if smoking a joint. Peter laughs and then becomes serious. "Innocence is always the most difficult thing to believe," he tells us. The song was for children and all speculation about drug metaphors are flat-out wrong.

Hollis introduces me to everyone at the table, explaining that I'm living with her and Jerome for a few months. She touches my hand softly and her bright blue eyes peer into mine. She doesn't even have to ask. I nod; I'm okay and we both smile. Jerome blows me a gentle kiss. I sit at the table for a while and only when I feel my hands begin to shake do I excuse myself. Peter turns to me. He has not even had a chance to get to know me, he says. Will I stay for a few more minutes? I move near his chair. I crouch next to him and he asks outright why I'm living here. He's gentle and kind and I speak without shame or uncertainty. His eyes grow soft as I talk. He puts a hand gently on my head and leans in. "Oh, you poor girl," he says. "My God, my God, my God. Those things are a horror. They are a *horror*." And the compassion in his voice is a buoy big as a house. I hold on to it as I ready myself for bed. Hours later, I hold it when the night claws open and my stomach seizes. The next morning I keep it close as I pull on my soft pants and drive to the grocery store.

That night, I sing "Puff the Magic Dragon" to Chloe. I sing it to her every night for the next year. I wrap the song around me and every time I sing it, I cry. I'm slowly learning to hold the buoy for myself, to let go of shame and touch the tear-streaked face of my own innocence.

# HUNCHED AND COCKY

## June 2012

SUMMER PASSES AND I COME OUT, blinking in the harsh light. It's been just over six weeks and I'm down to 45 milligrams of Valium. In the morning and at night I feed my children. In the afternoons I curl into a ball and wait out the pain. I ask Matt if it gets harder as you go down. He writes, "Yeah. For me, it did—I won't lie. What often happens is that the symptoms become more prolific for a time, with good days outnumbered by the bad as you get lower in dose and your receptors fight for equilibrium." So I buckle in. Every two weeks I drop my dose and within days I'm hunched. I stay hunched for five or six days, at which point I swing up to what feels like a mild flu. No biggie. Then I drop again.

Ivy and another friend have been sending me letters through the mail. Ivy's still in Salt Lake, only fifteen minutes from the house, but I never see her. I hardly see anyone. It's too painful to try to be normal, to manage the withdrawals that can roar to life within seconds. She says I'm sequestered like a monk. She writes on beautiful handmade paper. I still can't read well, so I put the letters on my nightstand and rub them with my fingers. I know Ivy has pulled away and I don't blame her. We were friends before the *Wasatch Journal* and became very close as colleagues.

We had dinner parties together and were consistent advocates for each other's work. Now we struggle because that life is gone. Sean and I don't see friends, we don't go to dinner parties or barbecues where the kids would play hide-and-seek and stumble through the backyard. We don't hang out on porches or go to birthday parties. Sean works and hikes and I've pulled myself into a cocoon of fire and no one knows what to do.

I ask Sean if we can go to counseling. "We need help," I say. "This is a prolonged sickness, and we need support." What I don't say is I can't feel love anywhere between us and this scares me. He says he'll go if I find someone, so I ask around and find Dr. Bruce. We go, and Sean sits braced. Dr. Bruce is a kind man, a big teddy bear with a razor-sharp intellect. After telling him about the past few months, he tells us that at the previous night's parenting class, the one he's been teaching for years, the subject of benzodiazepines just popped up. Out of nowhere, someone asked, "Is Ativan addictive?" Dr. Bruce laughs. Sean and I laugh. Ha. Oh, the hilarity of tragedy. And I can laugh because, although it's shredded my life, I'm several months into my detox and I've become just the slightest bit cocky about what a great patient I am.

*Is Ativan addictive?*

*Just a smidge more than heroin, but, hey, everyone's doing it.*

The therapy session feels okay. Sean is able to say that there's no space for *him* to feel sick and exhausted and I'm able to hear that. Dr. Bruce talks about the importance of staying connected, of having dates so we can remember we care for each other. We've gone through this before, but after three or four dates we forget or push it off, getting consumed with the overwhelm of our lives. Dr. Bruce emphasizes that on my good days we need to try to *connect*. If we simply endure, we're done for.

Sean and I go to a cheesy sports bar after therapy. We go out onto the patio because the televisions that loom in every corner feel like they're crawling over my body. The lights are bright, the images gross and sharp and fast. I know this hypersensitivity is part of the detox.

I'm okay with it. I've got the formula. I know how to deal with the withdrawal symptoms when they come on. Rage? Walk your ass off. Anxiety? Walk your ass off. Nausea? Walk your ass off. Then sleep. And eat as much as you can manage.

We sit. The patio is quiet except for the two bearded men huddled in the smoking cage that juts off at the corner of the back patio. We talk. We laugh. We discuss the insanity of social networking when we can barely manage the minutiae of our daily lives. "I'm flooded," Sean says. "The media, the networking, all of it. I just want to sit and feel what silence is like again." I agree.

We pay the bill and I go into the brightly lit corrugated aluminum stalls of the bathroom. This is when I realize I've forgotten to pick up my prescription. I'm out of the drug I hate, and I panic. I run out of the bathroom. I run out of the cheesy, hallucinatory sports bar. I'm out on the street. There's nowhere to go. It's nearly 10:30 p.m. The pharmacy is closed.

*Is Ativan addictive?*

If I don't get my little white pills, it's likely I'll have a seizure. It's that simple. You won't die from heroin withdrawal. You won't die from meth withdrawal. You won't die from opiate, pot, or antidepressant withdrawal. But benzodiazepines? Ativan? Yes, you can die. Just like that. Seizure. Brain goes ballistic. I've been cocky and now I'm terrified. If the benzos were human, they'd laugh. They'd say, *Thought you had us under control, babe? No go. We've still got your brain in the palm of our hands. We can crush you. Remember that.*

I call Jerome, who recognizes the terror in my voice right away.

"What's wrong?"

I babble. He calms me, says to find a twenty-four-hour pharmacy and he'll call in my dose for the night. I can't imagine what would happen if Jerome wasn't a psychiatrist whom I could call. What happens to other people who forget or take the wrong dose or think they can just stop taking the medication? I'm nearly sick in the parking lot.

Sean and I go to Walgreens and stare at the wall-to-wall plastic toys made in China. I pace back and forth in an aisle stocked with box after box of diet supplements, pregnancy tests, and condoms. Any sense of connection with Sean has been eclipsed by my burning terror about getting the Valium. My terror is a massive sun, a core-collapsed supernova consuming the whole sky.

By 11:00, I have my little white pills. Seizure averted. But I'm shaken. I forgot how I'm still subjugated, my brain trying hard to remember how it regulates things, since the benzos have slipped in and have been whispering *Hush* for so long. I'm so jacked up with adrenaline by the near miss I barely sleep that night. But I'm alive. I may be sleepless, but I'm alive. That counts for something.


IT'S JULY, AND it feels so good to stand next to the stage, watching incredible poets and storytellers gather a crowd at the Utah Arts Festival. I've always loved the sudden quiet, the way the crowd moves in tighter to hear amid the sonic interplay between various stages. And it's a little money. I feel good about contributing even a small amount. Sean has been stressed about being the sole provider, and while I think we're okay, I've been racked with guilt about not contributing more. So I stand and smile at the festival. I've walked and slept to keep the withdrawals at bay, but it's over 100 degrees out and the noise and basic interaction of boisterous humans is more than I can take. I read onstage at 4:00 p.m. and my knuckles go white against the mic. *It's good I'm a poet*, I think. *People will see my shaking and say the poets are tragically sensitive*. Back at Jerome and Hollis's house, my nose bleeds a thick red line for hours. It's a river, an ocean.

Last night I dropped my dose again. No sleep. I feel hideous. When I get up to take the kids to day care, they are like little demons. Chloe bites Finch, who just howls and crawls to the door to get Papa, who left for the job site at 7:00 a.m.

I swore to Sean after the festival that I'd do no more art shows, no more performances, no more anything but detoxing until my brain is mine again. It's a brutal catch-22. Performance and writing and art are my soul work, my love, the place I'm gifted and in my joy pocket. But I can't do it.

I MAKE A list of the things that sustain me; the things of Beauty. On the bad days I read it. It keeps me from spiraling too deep into the dark. It keeps me looking up.

1. *Sharon and her desire always to be kind. The innumerable loads of laundry she washes and folds without complaint.*
2. *Mom flying out for the weekends and sitting with me every other month even though she's broke.*
3. *Hollis and Jerome and the lilac and butter room.*
4. *Hollis and Jerome and the love so thick you could paint it on the walls.*
5. *Chloe's little-girl voice singing "Puff the Magic Dragon."*
6. *Finch hooting at 6:00 a.m.*
7. *Chloe saying, "Shake my groove thing."*
8. *Matt Samet, who is a goddamn rock star.*
9. *Dr. James, who swears he will get me off this shit.*
10. *Sean for keeping the lights on despite the fact we're crumbling.*
11. *Neff's Canyon, which lets me pound my rage into its soil.*
12. *Comedy Central.*
13. *Watching* Glee, *which helps me get my peace on.*
14. *The swallows that come at night and do their velvet curtain dance in the sky.*
15. *The sky with colors of Beauty: tangerine dream, butter coral, burnt blues.*

I look at this list and realize how lucky I am. I know what's happening. I know what to expect. I have some lanterns in the dark. One month into my taper down, when I was hunting for books, articles, anything that could give me information about the history and use of benzodiazepines, I found Robert Whitaker's book *Anatomy of an Epidemic: Magic Bullets, Psychiatric Drugs, and the Astonishing Rise of Mental Illness*, published in 2010. The book is an investigative journalist's exploration into all kinds of psychiatric drugs, but there is a long chapter on benzos. I learn that Valium was the bestselling drug in the Western world between 1968 and 1981, until magazines such as *Vogue*, *Ms.* magazine, and *Time* began running articles that claimed it was worse than heroin. I learn that Valium's fall from grace was rapidly remedied when Xanax—a much faster and more potent version of Valium—was brought to market to treat the newly identified "panic disorder" as described in the *Diagnostic and Statistical Manual of Mental Disorders*, fourth edition (*DSM-IV*).

Whitaker says that once benzos were marketed as a treatment for a mental illness, their place in the prescriptive cornucopia of pills for human maladies was solidified. Americans, it appeared, were plagued with panic, and Xanax and Ativan were the cure. And it's no wonder they seemed like sunshine, like a little bit of pharmaceutical magic. For those suffering acute anxiety or insomnia, the drugs are immediate and potent. According to Dr. James, emergency room patients suffering from grand mal seizures are given an injection of 2 milligrams of Ativan to stop the seizure in its tracks. This is the dose Dr. Amazing started me on. The wild run of the brain hits a massive pharmaceutical wall. But study after study show that while this drug is truly amazing for situational intervention—when one truly needs a hammer, say—its efficacy wanes after a week. After six weeks, many find little to no positive effect. But at six weeks of consistent use, the likelihood that you're hooked is high. Stopping the pills after six weeks could mean a tidal wave of insomnia. Or anxiety. Or a little trip of a psychotic break. You could end up screaming the lyrics from Chris Cornell's song "Black Hole Sun" from a rooftop or walking into a dark field where you decide to end it all.

Despite the darkness of all this information, I realize it's not the first time America has heralded a drug only to find it horribly destructive. It helps me to understand these things. Understanding our history of overprescribing makes me feel less alone somehow. There's a pattern of human confusion, a tendency I can wrap my mind around. From cocaine toothache drops to opium for bowel problems and menstrual problems, we've walked into dangerous waters before with our tinctures. But with each new medicine gone bad, it seems to require massive death and suffering before our miracle drugs are viewed with any real clarity. Opioids are the most recent of our deadly drugs, and it took an incredible uprising of those who had lost someone to bring the addiction and overdose potential to public awareness. Benzos are the next in line. I just happened to be in that line. And now I'm trying to get out.

I pray that soon I will eat and sleep again like a normal person. Because I want to be part of the tide that shifts awareness about these drugs. I want to survive so I can say, *Yes, it's hard to imagine, but could we have imagined thalidomide? Could we have imagined Nembutal, the barbiturate that was marketed as a suppository for nervous children? Could we have imagined that our chill pills could slowly dismantle our brains?*

I'M DOWN TO 19 milligrams of Valium. I've been seeing Dr. James once a month since I began my taper. I make the long drive to South Jordan and sit in the waiting room in front of the flat-screen TV and pretend I'm just someone with a cold, a little virus, nothing big. People come in and sit around me, always leaving at least one empty seat between us. We have our secrets. We stare at our shoes or the Disney movie that dances on the screen at the front of the room. When the nurse with the blond ponytail calls one of our names, we gather our things quickly. We smile small smiles and rush through the door.

I wait for seventeen minutes in the little white room. By now I've read all the pamphlets on diabetes and lower back pain. I've looked through the cabinets and tried on the latex gloves that bunch around my tiny fingers like extra-large condoms. I think how helpful it would be to add some information about the high addiction potential for benzos to the pink and purple flyers.

I consider turning this idea into a blog entry for Robert Whitaker's website Mad in America. I wrote to him when I first got his book and he asked me to be a guest blogger. I've written three blogs so far and thousands of people have read them. I've posted the links on Facebook, hoping the information will reach someone who needs it. *Maybe I can write about the flyers*, I think. Pink with big black caution boxes. Maybe. After I get through this bout. I am moving through this detox with a fury of will. I've dropped my dose and held until I stabilized and then dropped my dose again. I was doing well with the pace of the taper, but three nights ago the insomnia and the stomach cramps became overwhelming. I stand in the little exam room and sit. I do jumping jacks. I begin walking the room in small circles, because I shake if I sit for too long.

Dr. James bursts through the door, ducking his head as he walks in.

"Melissa," he says, his voice exuberant. "How's it going?" He flops in the chair near the computer and runs a massive hand through his mop of red hair. He looks at me. "You okay?"

I stop walking and rock from one foot to the other. And then I begin crying.

"Okay," he says, sitting up. "Okay . . . hey, I'm here. Tell me what's going on."

I stop rocking and walk over to the chair in front of him. I sit as if the chair may have spikes. My thighs shake. I press my hands against my thighs. My hands shake.

"I stopped sleeping again," I say. "On Tuesday. I don't know what happened." I'm still crying. I'm sure the mascara I've put on to try to make me look more awake is running rivulets down my face.

"You've been sleeping okay until now?"

"Yeah. It was enough. But three days ago . . ."

"Stopped sleeping."

"Yeah."

"How many hours do you think?"

"Maybe two? Maybe three . . . one hour a night? I'm not sure."

"Okay. Listen, this happens. It's not uncommon. Your brain is just saying it needs more time to adjust. We can handle this." He hands me a tissue. "Okay?"

He's leaning forward, elbows on his knees. He's got a big oval belt buckle that says *Toro* in crimson letters with a silver glitter outline. I blow my nose.

"This is the worst, Dr. James. It's what I was scared of."

"We can handle this," he says again. "Listen, I'm going to give you a prescription for the antipsychotic Seroquel. Don't let that scare you. In low doses, all it does is knock you out. It'll help you get over this hump."

"I don't want to take another drug."

"I know you don't, but gutting it out at this point is going to make the detox harder. Trust me."

"Is it addictive?"

"Yes. But nothing like benzos. I promise."

I press the tissue up against my eyes. I want to disappear.

"I hate this . . . I really *fucking* hate this."

"I know. It sucks. But it *will* get better. I want you to hold your dose for another two weeks, maybe a month. Don't start tapering until you've got some solid nights of sleep behind you." He looks for my eyes. "You got me?" I nod. "Okay. Is Sean with you today or did you come alone?"

"I came alone," I say, and start laughing. "Oh my God, I'm so totally alone right now, it's fucking hilarious." I keep laughing, bending in half to put my hands on my knees. Sean gave up on therapy with Dr. Bruce after three sessions. He said Dr. Bruce liked me too much and that he acted like a "cheerleader." Sean never comes with me to my appointments. It's me alone in this dark forest with Dr. James. I stare at the carpet and something in me steels. I stand up, gathering myself. "I'll be okay, Dr. James, really. I'll slap myself before I drive."

Dr. James puts his hand on my shoulder. "Listen, Melissa, I want you to think of the Seroquel as part of your arsenal. It's fucked-up that you have to use drugs to get off drugs, but it's our best option. The most important thing is you'll sleep tonight. I promise."

"Okay," I say. "Okay. Thanks, Dr. James. I like your belt buckle. It's really beautiful." I start laughing again and then crying. "Oh my God, I'm losing it."

"Melissa," he says. "Look at me. Give it two nights. I promise you'll sleep."

Dr. James hands me my prescription for Seroquel and walks me to the exit.

"I really don't know what I'd do without you," I say. "I don't think I'd make it."

"You will," he says. "You *will* make it. I've no doubt, Melissa. You're a fighter."

# FIVE-FOOT DRAGON

*October 2012*

I'M SLEEPING AND HOLDING AT 18 milligrams of Valium. I join a support group, feeling weak and tired from this day after day of relentless detoxing. I know I need help. And after the second meeting, the social worker turned therapist pulls me aside. There are ten women in the group—some recovering alcoholics, some anorexic, some dealing with death—but it's me she's worried about. It's me she asks to speak to after the group ends for the night.

We've just finished our peace meditation and extinguished the candle. There's talk about loving and accepting yourself just as you are in the moment. The group shuffles out and the therapist says she's worried about me. She's a substance abuse counselor, she tells me. She holds support groups for people getting off meds up at University Psychiatric Hospital. She's checked with another friend who works with addictions, mostly anorexia, and they both agree there's no way my withdrawal should take more than two weeks. Four weeks max. We're standing in her office. Candles and little stones that say *peace* and *serenity* litter her desk. Books on anorexia and women who love too much sit on her bookshelf.

She looks me in the eye and says, "I think you're obsessed with your withdrawal. There's no way this should take so many months.

And I'm worried this doctor you're working with is taking you for a ride." She waits. I stand, glancing at her rocks, her books, her candles of peace.

In seconds, I'm a powder keg. I will rise up like a black fire and devour her. I speak slowly, my eyes burning a hole in her head. "My doctor is one of two addictionologists in Utah. He knows more about what benzos do in the brain than anyone I've ever met. I feel confident that he isn't, as you say, *'taking me for a ride.'* " My body feels huge and looming. I let the silence between us grow big. I stay. This woman, this peace-and-love therapist—I want to rip her throat out.

"I'll get you his number if you'd like," I say. I'm growing bigger; I'm twenty feet tall. I'll crack her skull between my fingers and wipe the gore all over her pretty candles. She turns, shuffles some papers on her desk. I continue: "I'm happy to have you share your concerns with him. And by the way, as a substance abuse counselor, I imagine you're familiar with the Ashton Manual?" I'm clipped and calculated. This woman lights my shame on fire with her judgment. I feel murderous.

The peace-and-love therapist turns to me. Her lips are thin. She says that, no, she's never heard of the Ashton Manual. And yes, I should bring Dr. James's number to the next meeting. She'll try to carve out time to call him. She's concerned. Conversation over. I stand looming, watching her move papers into tight piles. After a minute I turn my dragon body and walk out.

And a week later Sean's sister in Idaho calls. When she was younger, she had some issues with drugs. This, apparently, gives her the tremendous insight that I am an addict, that Sean and his mother are "enabling me," and that I'm taking everyone for a ride. *Perhaps people who have had issues with drugs are the most judgmental*, I think. And then: *No, this is not the truth.* The truth is that some people are just assholes. And in this moment, my husband is also an asshole and complicit, because he delivers the news of his sister's sermon, her belief that I am fucking with them, as if she's written it out for him word for word. He's just telling me what she said, he repeats, his eyes flat, lips anemic. It's as if he's holding the poster board so he can be mute and his sister can say what he wishes he could say to me. I'm not at all sure how to receive this sermon delivered by proxy. "It's just what she said," he repeats for the third time, as if washing his hands of the whole thing.

And I don't know what to do with this indirect criticism offered as tag team by brother and sister. Because there is no to-my-face accusation. There is no *You're weak and a coward and you don't fool us with your story, you little maggot. Get home and take care of your children.* Honestly, I'd prefer this, because we could fight like proper dogs and tear each other open and then sob together huddled on the floor. But this aggression is at my back, and when I spin around, Sean tells me he doesn't understand why I'm so upset. It's no big deal.

Sean adds that now neither of his sisters feel they can talk to me again. His other sister, who lives here in Utah, is a pharmaceutical representative. One of my recent blogs refers to the record-setting $2.3 billion payout the pharmaceutical giant Pfizer made in 2009 for fraudulent drug marketing. I state that it was the largest health care fraud settlement and the largest criminal fine of any kind ever. My blog has nothing to do with Sean's sister, but I think she feels attacked. I'm shocked at the heat of judgment and crushed because not only did Sean not defend me, he delivered the news as if throwing darts while sipping a beer.

Despite all of this, Sean wants me back home. He doesn't say this, isn't direct in this way, only asks why I still need to be at Hollis and Jerome's after so many months. I'm halting, unsure of what to say, because the answer seems so obvious. I have not yet crawled out of this hellhole. I am in it every day and every night and I pull myself out to drive down and make breakfast or dinner, but it hurts every single day. Doesn't he understand this? Can't he see I'm still losing weight, that my ribs and hips make hard angles through my skin? Can he see me at all?

We talk in the bedroom and I remind him of all the withdrawal symptoms. I think that if he hears, it will make them real again. I realize how intangible it is, especially with me gone much of the day. I point out that between the two doctors working to help me, we've been given the time frame of nine months to two years for me to get off. He *knows*, he says sharply. He was *only asking*. And then he turns his back. I'm hollowed out by his dismissal.

And sometime later—a day? a week?—I'm in the grocery store with my cart full of pancake mix and milk, diapers and shampoo. In the cereal aisle, standing near the loaves of bread, is one of my old yoga teachers. I remember taking classes with her when I was pregnant and have always admired her soft blond curls, her yogic purpose. She greets me and fixes me with soft eyes. "Hello, Melissa," she says. "How *are* you?" The air fills with a strange, false feeling of friendliness complemented by her buttery yogic smile. I deflect. I talk about the heavy lifting of motherhood and how overjoyed I am that Chloe can sing "Puff the Magic Dragon" with me every night.

She cocks her head slightly. Our carts are lined up head to head in the aisle.

"I saw some of your blogs on Facebook," she says. "About your addiction." Her head shifts again. "Are you getting help with the cravings?"

"Cravings?" My jaw hangs on its hinges. "I'm sorry?"

"It must be hard."

I want to puke in her mouth. I want to punch her soft yoga face. This woman has clearly not read my posts. She saw the words "drugs, addiction, and dependency" and that was it. I became a user, just another addict struggling for the high. The hairs on my arms stand up. "There are no cravings," I tell her. "These drugs are punitive. I took them for insomnia and then I was told if I stopped taking them I would have a seizure. Physical dependency," I say, "is different than addiction." I'm gathering steam. She's asked, and she has fixed me with her yoga eyes, and so I will tell her. I'll unleash about the narrative of cultural shame that surrounds the term "addiction." I'll tell her how far it is from what I know and experience. "Benzodiazepines are unlike any other drug. Dependency can happen in the space of a week," I say. I've written the blogs, I tell her, because these drugs need to have strict monitoring. There's so much misinformation and I want to inform, to educate. I'm a train. I'm crashing down the tracks. I'm running her over.

She uncocks her head and cuts me off, saying she must be going. She must not have expected a train. She pushes her cart past mine. It was good to see me, she says, throwing back a wistful smile. She wishes me the best of luck.

I'm left standing alone in the aisle, which seems to stretch for miles in either direction. I feel vacant and furious. I feel sick at her inability, at our culture's inability, to see that we're making bombs with our drugs. These bombs go off in the brain, and the medical community has little real knowledge of what happens. Drugs go through the FDA with a wink as the trials that fail are filed away. This yoga woman saw me and saw the face of addiction as narrated by our culture. She had no knowledge of anything else.

I wonder how many of the people in this store are taking benzodiazepines. And of those who are, how many have laughed about it, made jokes about their chill pills, their Xanny bars and party candy, without having any idea that these same pills can slowly dysregulate the brain. How many could imagine that their emerging digestive problems, muscle aches, unexplained increases in anxiety or insomnia, were a result of the drugs they were taking? How many got diagnosed with irritable bowel syndrome, fibromyalgia, chronic fatigue, or a host of slippery neurological disorders? How many were prescribed pills and more pills to combat these ghost ailments? This is the big secret I want to scream in this woman's face: these pills are dismantling people slowly—so slowly, they imagine it's anything but their happy pills.

I remember the night I read the manual put together by Dr. Heather Ashton. The benzo.org.uk site posted innumerable research articles about what she and her colleagues called "protracted with-drawal symptoms." Outside the known realm of anxiety and insomnia, people in benzo withdrawal often get hit with perceptual symptoms (tingling, numbness, pain in the limbs), motor symptoms (pain, weak-ness, tremors, shaking attacks, jerks and spasms), and gastrointesti-nal symptoms that can be boiled down to feeling like your stomach has turned into a painful, inflatable aquarium. According to Ashton, these symptoms "may last at least a year and occasionally persist indefinitely." If I went to a doctor with complaints of numbness or weakness, electric shock sensations and tremors, they'd likely suspect multiple sclerosis or some other neurodegenerative disorder. If I told them I couldn't eat because my stomach cramped and burned, they'd look toward Crohn's disease or irritable bowel syndrome. If I hadn't discovered what was happening, I could be on a terrifying medical track or on terrifying new medications meant to remedy a disorder that was never a disorder at all.

I'm alone in the aisle with my heart thumping a heavy beat in my chest. Fluorescent lights blaze overhead. Music drones on at a calcu-lated, cheery frequency. A small child begins crying several aisles over, her howls lifting up and filling the air over my head. Where is Beauty at a time like this? I feel dismissed, cast aside with a practiced yoga smile and yoga eyes. I know people might see me as an addict, but to come face-to-face with it, despite my attempts to get the word out, is a reality that steals my breath. I feel punched in the chest and shame coats me like a sickness.

# GIANT BLACK WALL

# OF DESTRUCTION

*December 2012–May 2013*

FINCH, NOW FOUR YEARS OLD, IS kicked out of day care. We knew it was coming but I'd prayed that it would work for a few more months, just enough for ten more milligrams, but Finch's limits with language and his constant bolting from the classroom leave the teachers exhausted. We meet on a Friday in a conference room upstairs. The director tells us how hard they've tried. They put him in a room with younger kids a month ago, and when that didn't work, they tried him with the older kids. They installed a baby gate to block off the toddler room. Still, he evades them. He doesn't nap and doesn't understand their protests when he throws things off the shelves. Much later, we'll get the diagnosis that Finch also has autism, but for now all we know is that he gets frustrated and hits himself in the head when his surroundings are overwhelming— the crash of children's voices, the commands to sit still, stand in line, button up. The teachers are near tears. They say they'll keep him through mid-December but after that there's nothing they can do. Sean and I sit in conference chairs across from them. The round clockface just over the doorway says three o'clock. Our time here is up.

We tell them how grateful we are. Our boy needs us now. We understand this. His difference is difficult and beautiful, and we feel lucky they've chased him down over and over since I started Dr. James's withdrawal regimen over six months ago. We had no idea it would be so hard. But it is. It's harder than any of us could have imagined.

Sean and I walk through the building to the parking lot. Sean walks ahead of me. The sky is dark over the mountains, the trees spidery. We stand next to Sean's truck and talk about what we're going to do. The immediate answer is obvious: I have to move back to the house we call home.

"I'll start packing my stuff this week," I say.

"Okay," Sean says. "Sounds good."

"Shouldn't take much. I just have clothes and books and shampoo, stuff like that."

"Yeah."

"Um. So maybe next Monday? I'll bring my stuff back to the house?" He nods.

"Okay." We stand for a few minutes as drops of rain begin falling. "So what about your mom?"

"What about her?"

"Is she going to stay with us? Keep helping? I still have fifteen milligrams to go. I don't know if I can do it without someone to help with the basics. I just . . . It could take another six months."

"Six months?" Sean's furious. "How can it take six months? You've gotten off, what, over thirty milligrams in about six months? How can it take *six more*?"

"It just . . . Dr. James says it could. And any kind of stressor is like adding more weight to a thin sheet of ice and I'll stop sleeping again and . . . Sean . . . the GABA receptors in my brain are trying hard to recover but we just *don't know* how long it will take them to rewire. You have no idea how desperate I am to feel normal, to feel human again."

"I thought you were getting better."

"I'll start to get better when I'm finally off. Fifteen every day is still pretty high. A typical dose is maybe five," I add. "On occasion."

Sean stares across the parking lot, his mouth and eyes hard.

"And that could be another six months," he says without looking at me.

"Yeah. I mean, I just don't know."

"I think her mom wants her to come to Kentucky."

This is how Sean says *No*. He cannot say it himself, but he can say it by proxy.

"Oh. She usually goes to Kentucky in the winter, doesn't she? To be with her mom?"

"Yeah."

"Can't she stay a little longer?"

Sean opens the door to his truck.

"Her mom needs her," he says, "in Kentucky."


Dr. James tells me that the last five milligrams can be the hardest. Who knows why? He recommends that with the increase in stress—the return to home and the return to full-time homemaker—I should go as slowly as possible. And there's something called titration. It involves crushing up the Valium and dissolving it in water or milk so I can measure my dose in milliliters. You can buy beakers online, he tells me; eBay is great. And there are plenty of YouTube videos on Valium titration techniques, right next to the innumerable pages of videos people have posted about their experiences trying to get off benzodiazepines. Maybe I'll fold little socks and watch. I'll make menus for the week and precise titration schedules that will drop my dose in barely perceptible milliliters. I tell myself it will work. Who cares if it takes six or eight more months? I'll be home with my boy and we'll rock this titration thing.

We wave goodbye to Sharon, who flies away to Kentucky on a Wednesday. The kids and I make a book with pictures and lists of

"Things We Love About Nana." She's been with us eight months. And then she's gone. Sean seems briefly happy, relieved to have me back and his mother off to care for someone else. I make an effort at normalcy. I look up meat loaf recipes and do research on how to potty train someone with Down syndrome, which, according to some sources, could take up to a year. I start a WordPress blog to write anything and everything. It's one of many attempts I keep making to find my way back to myself. I write about my efforts to potty train Finch, comparing waiting with him on his little plastic dinosaur potty to a very dull period of French literature. I write about the day Chloe holds my face in her hands and says, "I eat you, Mama." I write about my fury and about the pruning of the brain receptors that happens with long-term use of benzos. I write about "Embracing Joy as a Moral Obligation." I try to harness myself with my own words.

Sean shuffles around in his office and we sleep in the same bed. We're normal. We're just like our neighbors, people who hold barbecues and talk about their mortgages. We watch sports! Go Utes! Go Patriots! I count pills at night but I'm good now. I'm close enough. We tell friends that come spring I'll be right as rain.

The long days of watching Finch run from door to door in the house, trying to get the doors unlocked, hurts. And wanting him to understand how to pee in the potty hurts. And when we go to the grocery store—where he kicks and yells to get out of the shopping cart, leaving me gripping the handle—despair and hopelessness are like a cocoon of spun glass inside me. And then Chloe gets the stomach flu. And it's three days of holding her limp body on the couch with Tupperware at the ready and her crying, "Mama, Mama," and fire ants everywhere under my skin. And I could maybe take it if the unsaid thing—that Sean and I are broken—didn't pulse through the house. The tension of our fracture hits me like a flung stone, and I can't get rid of it.

The first week home, despite keeping my dose stable, my intestines shut down. I can't eat. I can't shit. I barely sleep, an indicator that my brain is in hyperdrive and the GABA receptors are not doing well. Most nights I spend huddled on the couch in the living room. I tell Sean I've lost four more pounds, bringing me to what I weighed when I was eleven years old. When I say I feel worse than I've felt in months, he answers, "No you don't."

And I realize he's hit his limit. He hit his limit so long ago. He takes long hikes all through the fall. He goes to southern Utah and camps alone. He hikes almost fourteen miles to Mount Timpanogos, one of the highest peaks in the Salt Lake Valley, only to collapse in sobs at the top, undone in the thin air. He tells me this later, as if in surprise. He's living half a life and stays zipped inside himself, allowing his fury and grief out only after he's exhausted his body and only when alone. Emotional exhaustion burns like a torch in the muscles. We can't take any more. For a while we ignore the suffocation that has become our marriage. We pretend the light-headedness, the numbness, is an aberration. We do this together because to acknowledge the death of our relationship is a brutality we can't bear. I continue to make meat loaf and quiches, pancakes and oatmeal. We lie like husband and wife and I crush pills into little beakers filled with milk late at night. The fever stays close and it takes me another six months to go from 15 milligrams to 5.

ONE DAY IN early May, I take my wedding ring off, drop it into a pretty box, and put it on a shelf in the closet. I don't know what makes this day different from the rest. Perhaps I, too, have simply hit my limit. I don't have the voice to say I feel there's nothing left in our marriage. But I can untether myself from the ring. I can pull the symbol off.

The following week Sean loses his ring in someone else's yard. He jokes he must have dropped some of the baby weight because the ring was there and then it was gone. It's buried deep in the dirt near the lettuce, he says. Maybe it's lying atop a mound of compost. He doesn't know. We make jokes. We take it lightly. It's no big deal. We can buy new ones.

As I begin tapering down from 5 milligrams, my body bucks. Every night, I crush 5 milligrams of Valium and put the powder into a 100-milliliter beaker with milk. I drink 98 milliliters and dump the remaining 2 milliliters. This is micro-tapering. It's as slow as you can go. I'm alone in the kitchen with the light casting shadows in the corners. Sean is always somewhere else. He does not want to watch me do this. After two weeks of crushing 5 milligrams of Valium into milliliters, I am down from 100 to almost 60 milliliters. I drink 60 milliliters of Valium milk and dump 40. I don't know quite how this translates into milligrams. All I know is the feeling of flu in my body is constant. Sean and I try to have sex and my skin burns when he grabs my ass, my neck. It hurts when he pulls me to him. Sean touches me and my body is a cold, sick fire. I go through the motions hoping for relief, that blessing of skin, but it eludes me. After having sex, Sean rolls over to sleep and I tuck my body into a small ball. I will endure this cold fire for as long as I can, but I'm getting tired.

# NORMAL

*Late May–August 2013*

I'M WIDE-AWAKE, BLINKING AND SHADING MY eyes against the sun when it happens. I'm driving the kids to their Saturday morning tumbling class at Little Gym, an international franchisor of infant- and child-oriented fitness gyms. They throw themselves onto blue and red mats. They pretend to be butterflies. I'm the quiet mother, the one who always seems propped against the wall, the one who wobbles.

We're driving on a side street, just two blocks from the main intersection, when my vision goes blurry. Lines on the road double and shift. Then, out of nowhere, the cars and road disappear and I'm driving in inky darkness. Eyes wide-open, I blink and blink. Finch hoots behind me. Chloe feels a shift. "Mama?" Sounds of traffic become acute: a car moving past, a horn. My hands grip the nubbed leather of the steering wheel, terrified. I go all at once electric, adrenaline surging. My feet tap the brake and I swerve right, slamming my foot down when I hear the crunch of gravel beneath the tires. A sharp horn. Someone yells for me to fucking watch it. Thirty seconds later, a lifetime later, my vision returns, blinks on in the bright light of day. I'm angled off the side of the road, inches from a white fence surrounding a square of green. Anyone could have been standing there when I swerved—a little boy or girl making chalk rainbows, writing their names on the sidewalk. Anyone.

THE NIGHT AFTER my vision goes black, I talk with Sean about temporarily stopping my taper. I've spent a year and a half clawing in the underworld, trying to get off the medication that I was on for a year and a half. I'm hovering somewhere near 4 milligrams of Valium and I'm so goddamn tired. Sean's happy. He just wants normal, he tells me. His season's starting to peak. He needs my support. We agree. I call Dr. James, who tells me to hold at 5 milligrams of Valium. A break from the grueling withdrawal will do me good. I can gain some weight. I can restart my titration in the fall.

And we do find a kind of normal. Every day, I take Finch and Chloe to the pool. I read them *The Cat in the Hat* and *Thomas the Tank Engine*. I wake up and stand. I walk to the park without folding. I shop at the grocery store without leaving my cart in the cereal aisle and fleeing in terror from the gore of fluorescent lights and the cacophony.

In August I start taking capoeira, a Brazilian martial art that looks as much like dance as anything. My friend Sedina and her husband, Dave, have practiced capoeira for years and they encourage me to come to classes with them. The classes are physical and acrobatic, and they feel like an apt metaphor for my life right now: fighting that's equal play and dance. It's beautiful and fierce and, what's better, it makes me feel normal. I wish I could bring this into my relationship with Sean. I keep hoping the tension between us will resolve, but it feels like it's hardened. It's heartbreaking after everything we've been through, but even here I have to let go. We've become testaments to each other's loneliness. I remind myself that loss isn't something one can control.

When the evening hits the magic hour and gold lights the mountains, I bring Chloe outside and teach her the names of birds. She's almost four now and loves sitting with me on the porch, pointing to the trees and the sky: sparrow, woodpecker, robin, finch. "Yes, honey," I say, "we named your brother after a bird."

I send Matt emails about the beautiful momentum of normalcy. He writes that I'm a warrior and that my brain will continue to get better. Sometime in the middle of the summer I get a side gig writing fundraising proposals for a nonprofit. I have Chloe help me work on a collage of birds and antique wallpaper. I almost forgot how good it feels to feel good. But something has changed. The great humility of this dependency has brought me to my knees. And it's on my knees that I've learned that mothering is about holding my own hand and wiping my own tears. Out of the deepest loneliness I've ever felt, I've discovered an intimacy with my own fears and insecurities. After so many times clutching my stomach as it seizes or watching Sean walk away from me when I feel I can barely stand, I've discovered my own strength. I feel like a house that has somehow remained standing in the wake of a massive fire. In having my life annihilated, metaphorically burned nearly to the ground, I've gained a new one. A new coal has been lit. I can feel its warmth spreading, sparks jumping to light in my body.


A TORNADO HIT Moore, Oklahoma, today, a town over one thousand miles away. It's been all over the news: talk of unstable air mass, deep-layer wind shear, and supercells. I don't know what any of this means. It sounds technical and scary and it boils down to the perfect storm turning the sky purple, then pea green, and then a tornado drops in like some god's hand pumping the air into a two-hundred-mile-per-hour frenzy. The twister was on the ground for forty minutes, crashing through seventeen miles of highly populated Oklahoma landscape. It's hard for me to imagine. Some of the people interviewed—always standing knee-deep in the remains of their shredded paper homes—said the tornado resembled a "giant black wall of destruction."

I've never been to Oklahoma, but I wonder how these people will put their lives back together. How does anyone reclaim a life after it's been obliterated? Do you sift through the wreckage? Do you fill out forms and cling to hope, or do you just call it, walk into the distance, and start fresh?

I watch the video footage for two days straight. I think of the French philosopher Simone Weil, whom I've been trying to read and who was, I believe, as smart and as kind as all the Greek philosophers I've read. Even Albert Camus thought she was "the only great spirit of our times." Weil's *First and Last Notebooks* talks about the relationship between our physical and spiritual suffering. She wrote the last book in the middle of World War II, while dying from tuberculosis. *She was a gentle Buddhist*, I think. She talked about the resistance to suffering as being a "second arrow" to the soul. The initial suffering is the first arrow. The second and perhaps more painful is the resistance to the things that hurt. *Don't stiffen*, I imagine her saying. *Lean in. Even the hard parts are Beauty. Even that is part of the awe of living.*

Sean isn't interested when I tell him the tornado hit the elementary school. He tells me the Midwest is used to tornados. People will just pick up and rebuild. I tell him the theater and the cemetery were uprooted. "Can you imagine? Corpses flying through the air? Theater chairs ripped up and flung into a field miles and miles away?" Homes were flattened, I say. Tank trucks were tossed into the air like confetti. I don't say that Weil believed that the love of our neighbor in all its fullness simply means being able to say, *What are you going through?* I don't tell him I wish I could go there. I wish I could hold their hands.

"It happens," he says, brushing off my comments as if Oklahoma were just another foldout brochure in a glossy travel magazine.

"But this one was bad," I say. "This one was really, really bad."

The next night Sean and I fight. We're on our way to have dinner with Sedina and Dave, whom we haven't seen since my fortieth birthday party. Sedina and I were pregnant with our boys together, had even put together a poetry performance when we were nine months pregnant. They're friends I've had since before I met Sean. To him they're peripheral. To me they represent who I used to be. I tell Sean I have some editorial work to do on Sunday, a brief gig, but it's money. I haven't worked at all through my withdrawal, so this feels like a chance to contribute financially. I want to do this. Sean gets tight as a drum and says he wanted to take a hike that day. We spiral. We're assholes. We're stupid and ugly and flying down the road blind and there's nothing stopping us. It's one of those arguments that's like stepping on an anthill. One step and ants are a river up my calves to my thighs. I open my mouth to say *Wait* but ants swarm into my mouth. The argument doesn't end; we simply arrive in the new driveway of Sedina and Dave's new house and Sean stares ahead at the new garage, the fresh paint. After several minutes, still facing the garage, he says, "I'm sorry you're so frustrated."

To which I respond, "Thanks." And we sit there, the words dead animals between us. We open our doors and get out of the car. I wipe my mouth on my sleeve. Sean strides in front of me to ring the doorbell. "Hello, hello—so good to see you." Kisses and wide smiles. We create the illusion that everything is fine. No blood here, no shards of glass, no ship sinking into black water. We are so good at this. We've done it for so long.

Two days later, when Sean is out for a hike, Ann comes over. She's not helping regularly the way she used to. Her fibromyalgia has kicked up, so she's often in pain. I'm grateful to have her come over whenever she can. I take an hour to retreat to the backyard, overgrown but full of dark purple irises and high grasses. I begin writing and my sadness pours onto the page. Sean and me, lost. This grief rises inside of me. I'm consumed with loss. I look toward the sky as I always do. Two robins play, tussling for a moment, and then catapult toward the large trees in the yard before flying up to play again. This is what I want. This is what I keep hoping Sean and I will find again, but for now, there's only grief. It's grief born out of the knowledge that we won't survive this. I feel almost sure, but I will circle back through denial for a while. There's no forcing the seed of knowing to open. I know this. I know that I'll circle and wail and try until a clear knowing rises up. But for now, a heat of sadness burns in my chest. We've tried so hard, both of us. But sometimes the very act of survival breaks things.

# THE INSOMNIA TAPES

*November 2013*

WHEN THE PRODUCER FROM ABC EMAILS me, she tells me she has a nephew who was prescribed benzos. She doesn't give me details but tells me she was shocked by what happened to him. She wants to set up an interview as soon as possible. I've been holding at 5 milligrams of Valium since the summer and haven't restarted my titration. The stress in the house is at a high pitch and I just can't face the despair of withdrawals right now. The first producer writes a few times and then tells me she has a family emergency. She's handing the story off to another freelance producer. A few days later, Len Goldstein emails. He tells me they need drama to move the story forward. They need an arc. They need anguish. Will I consent to doing a video diary, documenting going off the last five milligrams with a handheld camera?

I consider agreeing to the video diary for all of a day. Death is everywhere—why not capture it on film? Why not expose myself to enable the exposure of a great injustice? I talk to Hollis and she says she understands, but do I really want to throw myself back into the hellhole of benzo withdrawal? Now? With the distance between Sean and me feeling hopeless and permanent? Hasn't it all been too much? she asks. And isn't this exactly the kind of sensationalism I want to avoid?

And she's right, of course. Even if ABC comes, there's no guarantee they won't chop the diary into five seconds, and for what? I email Len and tell him I won't do the video diary. I say there are innumerable videos of withdrawals on YouTube. There are hundreds. They could get the okay to use them, but, to be honest, the videos aren't that remarkable. Anguish is quiet, I tell him. The people in the videos speak slowly, and urgency fills their voices, but there's no blood. There are no needles or smoke; there are people pacing and there are tics and tremors and the sense of unfathomable weight bearing down on them. He emails me the same day and says they need something to intersperse between sections of the interview. Do I have any pictures of myself tragically thin? Will I do a video diary of my lingering insomnia? I agree to the insomnia diary despite the fact my insomnia is now manageable. I've stabilized on 5 milligrams of Valium and I average about six or seven hours of sleep a night. Some nights are still raw, but after so long, I can take the occasional night of only two or three hours. The producer says he'll FedEx me an infrared camera. He wants me to use my iPhone to record myself at night. *Say it's 3 a.m. and how long you've been up*, he emails. *Say anything. We need to get working.* They want to air the piece in late December—early January at the latest.

When the camera comes, I set it up at the foot of the bed. I try to keep Sean out of the picture, but you can see bits of leg and an occasional arm. I film for five nights and have insomnia for two. The video is grainy and uninteresting. I get in bed and lie there. I toss. I sit up and stare into the distance, which I hope adds drama. I realize I'm trying to add drama, so I crawl out of bed for some water. I walk into the front room as I usually do. I return to bed and slump against the pillow with more vigor than usual. I'm trying to act tired. I'm acting haggard for ABC.

I email Len that the insomnia tapes are boring. He tells me not to worry, just keep taping. They can work with boring. One night I go into the bathroom and set up my iPhone so I can record myself in the mirror. I've just watched a clip of late-night talk show host and comedian Jimmy Fallon. I try to imitate his cool and after three or four takes I'm killing it. I perform what I call a "Hashtag Primer on Benzodiazepines" and send it to Len at 4:15 in the morning. He emails back saying I'm hilarious. Keep sending stuff. I know they'll never use it, but the night diaries have given me a creative vehicle to try to explain the savagery of benzodiazepines. I can make it funny. I can make it tragic and funny and poignant. I can make references to popular culture. I know the musicians who talk about Xanax and Klonopin. I know the Jon Stewart jokes. I know it all.

Night after night I send recordings and Len tells me that soon they'll fly in a correspondent. It's going to happen. I realize that I'm trying everything. I'm desperate to show people how horrific benzodiazepines can be, how they can shred your life into tiny, fragmented shards. I think if I can be funny, people will hear; if I can ache with honesty, people will hear. The truth is, I'm terrified they won't hear at all. I'm terrified they'll dismiss the whole thing as a medical anomaly or me as a Rolling Stones cliché, a mother's little helper who helped herself too much.

Sean and I argue about my being on television. I'm sitting on the bed. He's standing with his hand on the dresser and he says I want the limelight; I want my name ten feet tall and luminous. I tell him all I care about is saving other people from the hell realm of what we've gone through, but his fury is set loose and running, alternately hitting me over the head with a shovel and then himself. "You're an egomaniac," he says. "You're dynamic and great at a dinner table. I'm just a guy trying to raise two kids."

One night I bring up the idea of us separating. I'm sitting in the front room. Sean and I have put the kids to bed, and he comes and stands looking at me from the threshold between the kitchen and living room. Even now the distance between us feels physical. He stands in the doorway, not entering or exiting. We're existing in an in-between state and I can't stand it. I've thought of us separating for a long time, but I've never voiced it before tonight. "Maybe we could do a trial separation," I say. "Even if it's just for a while." I feel anguish like an anvil on my chest. "Sean, we've lost ourselves." The conversation goes nowhere because neither of us can take the final step. Sean says he's thought of it but can't face the immeasurable sadness of separation. I sit there watching his hands bracing his body in the doorway. "I know, I know," I say. "I'm so sorry," as if my despair can make it better, as if I can somehow obliterate the grief consuming our bodies.

When Christmas week comes, I convince Sean to give our relationship one last shot. It's my Elisabeth Kübler-Ross moment. I'm moving through the *denial* stage in the five stages of grief popularized by Kübler-Ross in the late 1960s. Maybe I'm in the *bargaining* stage. Hard to say, but I'm suddenly gripped by feeling that somehow, if we try hard enough, we can find our way back to each other. We sit in the office a few days before Christmas morning and I enthuse: "We can do this! I know we can." We both agree we'll do whatever it takes to make it work. It's been a disaster, a storm of magnificent proportions, but we can get to shore together, we say. We're giddy with the thought. It doesn't have to end. I believe this because it's the last tether I have. I've lost so much already. I want to believe that Sean and I can rebuild our house of love. We both want to believe.

Sean gets a big tree and Chloe helps put the little glass balls and gold ribbon on the lower third. I wind the ribbon through the upper portion of the tree and attach an assortment of red cardinals I find at a craft store. When we put on the lights, Finch loses his mind, pulling the lights off the tree and putting them into his mouth. We take turns distracting him and eventually he gets immersed in shoving anything he can find into the stockings I've set out on the couch. Later, I find a banana peel, a broken windup car, a roll of Scotch tape, and my phone stuffed into the stocking.

Ann comes over on Christmas morning. She sits in her chair in the kitchen with a big mug of coffee and we both remind Chloe and Finch they can't tear open the presents until *after* we eat the bacon omelets Sean has cooked. While we're waiting, the kids toddle over to the window in the living room and place their hands against the glass, peering out. There was a big snowfall overnight, so the yard is a soft and glittery pillow. The Christmas tree is lit up behind them with presents spilling from underneath in bright colors. I walk next to Finch and breathe on the window, taking his finger to trace the outline of a heart.

"Heart," I say, and he looks up at me, marveling, as if I made the curved lines appear out of thin air.

"Heart, Mama," he says. This beautiful boy. I realize that, rather than me teaching him *my* language, he's teaching me his. Rapture. Connection. These are the words and concepts that he speaks. He doesn't waste time with anything else.

After we eat and pick out the last bits of bacon for Finch, who would eat it all day, every day if he could, we move into the living room. I play Santa, handing out gifts while the kids tear at their packages. Chloe has started teaching Finch how to tear at the wrapping paper. Her fingers are more deft and he delights in holding the boxes while she rips the paper to ribbons. Sean and I sit close on the couch. My legs drape over his and his hand rests lightly on my thigh. I trace the line of his fingers. It all feels so good and so right. We are a family. We're having Christmas and there are no arguments, only the tearing of paper by small hands and the ecstatic glee as they find the rubber ball, the train set, the little green and blue elephants that stack like blocks.

Ann sits near the window. Chloe runs up to show her the colored markers she's just unwrapped. Ann oohs and aahs and Chloe drops markers at her feet. She runs back to the tree and looks at me expectantly. She wants more. She's in toddler heaven, tearing every package open and throwing ribbon and paper heedless into the air.

"I love Christmas," Ann says, smiling at Sean and me.

"Me too," I say, weaving my fingers between Sean's and snuggling closer. We're high on hope and the light of Christmas. There's so much beauty, so much tenderness. In the afternoon, Sean and I take the kids outside to build a snowman. I grab a scarf and a carrot. Finch and Chloe dive headfirst into the snow, delighting in the soft plumes surrounding them. Later, Ann makes hot chocolate and Sean and I put together Finch's train set. We get out the window markers and I draw an ocean, birds, and a sky. We erase it and I help Chloe sketch a house with flowers and stick figures. "Papa," I say, pointing to the tall figure. "Mama." We look out. We're creating a new life. Today is Christmas and we have the chance to create something entirely new. We will plant new seeds. We will regrow our roots together.

LEN GOLDSTEIN AND an LA correspondent will be here tomorrow. It's early January and I've sent innumerable recordings on my iPhone, recorded myself getting in and out of bed throughout the night and sent them as much information as I can on benzodiazepines. The warmth between Sean and me lasts all of a few days. We had Christmas. That was something. But by the next day a chill again fills the air between us. When I approach him with anything involving ABC, the cold turns icy. I tell him I still don't know what angle they're going to take. He asks no questions, just says he wants to be left out of the whole thing. Len tells me they'll film me for half the day and then film Dr. James. Dr. James will be their expert. He'll talk about the high addiction potential with benzos, how after two weeks you can be so hooked you'll have a seizure if you quit. And when they ask him whether benzos are recreational, he'll laugh. I can see him with his big hands explaining that while some people combine them recreationally with other drugs, for the most part people are simply following their doctor's orders. And if the doctor prescribes them for situational use, all is well. Occasional use doesn't foster addiction. But long-term prescribing by general practitioners has exploded up and up, normalizing their use and increasing the number of those who are unknowingly addicted.

He'll explain the typical scenario of someone running out of pre-scribed benzodiazepine and deciding to pick up their prescription in a few days. No big deal. But when they wake with chills, body tremors, nausea, they may think they have a terrible flu, a new viral epidemic that ravages the body and mind. They won't understand, at least ini-tially, that what they're feeling is the experience of being dope sick. There's no dopamine high with benzos, Dr. James will tell them, no body surge or superhero flush. You just feel like you're going to die if you don't take them. Dr. James's giant form will shift in the small, clean office chair. His red hair will blaze on the screen. He'll talk briefly about GABA receptors and his presence will be so big, so reliable, people will know there's something different going on here. I imagine him comparing the benzodiazepine epidemic with the opiate problem. Benzodiazepines, he'll say, are just as dangerous, but we're ten years behind in our understanding of them because they're so stealth. They're more complex, their action on the brain more devas-tating. Dr. James will make people understand that these little pills are killing people. He will make them understand. He's got to.

And then, without my pressing, Sean decides he's in. He agrees to be interviewed and feels okay about having the kids on camera. It'll be brief, Len promises. The kids will be the visual showing me as Mama. They'll do shots of me running down the street and typing on my com-puter. *She's a mother*, the images will say. *She's a writer and an athlete.* They'll take shots of the medicine cabinet. *And here*, the camera will say, *is her brain on her doctor's drugs*.

Since Christmas, there's been a hush between Sean and me. There's still so much unsaid. We've hidden our feelings and resentments under the proverbial rug. The benzo withdrawal was so acute, there was no room to put them anywhere else. And now the resentments and mis-understandings have become so big, we don't know where to start. We hope all our conflict and resentment will dissipate, but the feelings stay under that rug, a massive pile of hurt tripping us up. We walk the structure of our lives: shop for groceries, do the laundry, find the keys. There's thunder between us, but for now, we can ignore it. We have ABC coming. We can focus on that.

At 9:00 a.m. on Tuesday, Len Goldstein rings our bell. I'm wearing a periwinkle dress and gray boots with buckles on the side. I've taken a blow-dryer to my hair and it's long and straight, just like my mascaraed eyelashes. I open the door.

Len stands in the doorway chewing on his pinkie nail. He's average height, with circles under his eyes and kinky hair rising in puffs around his head.

"Melissa?" he asks.

"Who?" I say. I'm trying to be funny. I smile.

"Hey," he says, smiling. A pause. He appraises me. "You're shorter than I thought you would be."

Len walks through the door and looks around the living room. He appraises light and space. I shuffle my feet.

"Would you like some coffee?" I offer.

He shows me a half-empty bottle of Diet Coke. "I've got three of these," he says. "I'm good until lunchtime. Thanks." He looks me over again. "Good work with the dress."

Five minutes later a big white van pulls into the driveway. Two guys in jeans and T-shirts get out and haul in camera equipment. The front room fills up. They'll use two cameras simultaneously to film the correspondent and me.

"Cecilia will be here in fifteen minutes," Len tells the camera guys. "Have either of you worked with her?" The camera guys, whose names are Mike and Craig, shake their heads. "She covered the Fukushima disaster," he says, taking a swig of Diet Coke. "Better her than me," he adds before turning to me. "Hey, where are the kids?"

Sean is downstairs with Finch and Chloe. We agreed it was best to keep the kids out of the way until they were needed. All the chaos and equipment would be a bad combination for Finch, who'll want to pull out the plugs and yank on the cords for the tall lights. He'd have the whole setup on the floor and disassembled in three minutes flat.

I stare at the bulky black cameras on tripods—the entire room is filled with lighting equipment and microphones—and remember the film I put together when my mother was just a week out of rehab. I was skipping school for a long time and no one had said a thing. I went to a big California public high school and there were at least three hundred students in my senior class. It was easy for me to fall through the cracks. With so many students, they lost track and I knew how to work the system. I rerouted recorded calls the school made to our home and forged notes saying I'd been to the doctor. When I was a senior, my mother lost her job and was usually so drunk or high, she had no idea I'd skip school and take the bus to San Francisco. When she admitted herself into rehab, the news somehow got back to my school counselor.

Dr. Edmonds was compassionate and overworked. He had light hair and a ruddy face, and he liked me. Most of my teachers liked me, because I talked up a storm in class, whether I'd done the assignment or not. So after asking me a few questions about what I did in San Francisco—"Photo-essays on the homeless"—and talking to me about what I was doing while my mom was in the hospital—"Working at a café so there's food; reading this supercool biography of Jim Morrison"—Dr. Edmonds gave me a choice. I could do a project for each of my teachers and graduate or do nothing and not graduate. "We all know you're smart," he said. "But being smart isn't everything. State law requires you be in class. However, your circumstances are unusual . . ." And so I'd agreed. I spent hours working a script about alcohol and drug addiction. I included facts and figures. My boyfriend, Matt, played the part of the KQED newscaster, reading off worrisome statistics in front of a sheeted backdrop. And in between the newscast and the satire of a Dewar's Scotch commercial in which my brother played the Dewar's Scotch man, I interviewed my mother.

I don't remember much about what I asked her. I don't remember playing the video for the school. I do remember feeling detached and numb and later watching my biology teacher break down in sobs. "My husband," she said, pressing her hands against her face. "Oh my God." And I stood shuffling my feet in front of her desk, the room sickly sweet with the formalin used to preserve biological specimens. I didn't know what to say. I had no clue what I'd done. I knew I'd graduate with low marks, and my mother seemed fragile as china. Since she got out of rehab, I watched her cry and eat jelly beans and McDonald's fries all day. Beyond that, I was dazed and paralyzed with my heart wound. This was what brought me to art first. I had no name for what I was feeling, but art did. Art and poetry gave my wounds a home.

I walk downstairs to get the kids. Sean is watching *Sesame Street* with Finch on his lap and Chloe is coloring on the lime-green kiddie Ikea table I got when we moved in.

"Len wants to meet the kids," I say. "But there's a lot of equipment up there."

Sean glances up at me. He's not excited about having ABC here. He's enduring ABC, enduring me. He sighs. "Just bring Chloe. I'll stay here with Finch until they're ready to film. Having so many people upstairs will freak him out."

I consider this and decide Sean's right. The whole thing is bizarre—having people come in and take over part of your home so you can spill your guts on national television.

"Yeah," I say. "Good idea."

I bring Chloe upstairs and Len shows her the camera and tells her they're making a movie and she's going to be in it. She's shy but warms when he lets her touch the big camera and look through the lens. Len and I talk about the various scenes they want to film. They'll shoot me putting Chloe's pink, glittery high-tops on her feet. We'll try to get a shot with Finch. Maybe I can hold him so he doesn't knock over a camera. Maybe we can get a nuzzle. When Cecilia arrives, we'll do the interview and then move to the kitchen to interview Sean and me together. There will be shots of me on the computer and jogging down the street. Oh, and the medicine cabinet. How many meds do I take now just to sleep? And this is all to counter the damage done by the benzos, right?

Len gets his second Diet Coke out of the fridge as Cecilia arrives by taxi. She's long-legged and beautiful, with dark brown hair and dark eyes. I offer her coffee, which she accepts.

"I took the red-eye from New York yesterday and got the connecting flight from LAX this morning," she tells me. "I'm exhausted. But then," she says, smiling, "I'm always exhausted."

Chloe and I sit near the kitchen table as Len and Cecilia talk through the shots. They've worked together before. The camera guys stand in the doorway and wait. They've been contracted through a clearinghouse the major networks use. I start chatting with one of them. He's a climber and we know some people in common. He tells me he hates working for the networks but that it pays the bills.

Len turns to me.

"Okay," he says. "We're going to start with the high-tops. You two ready?"

We film for three hours. Scene after scene after scene. The interview between Cecilia and me is the hardest to set up. The lighting has to be just right, and we have that big window. Cecilia sits across from me with a big light shining on her face. I'm sitting on a stool with my hands between my legs.

"Just relax," she says. "We're just having a conversation—you and me."

She asks me to tell her what happened. When did I realize it was the drugs that were making me sick? How skinny did I get? And what happened during the blackout in the car? What about the time I collapsed in Chloe's room and had to crawl up the stairs? The sudden muscle seizures? She has a suitcase full of questions and is easy to talk to, even though I can see Len chewing his nails just four feet away.

I ask her if she's heard of the story of the boiling frog. She shakes her head.

"Okay," I say. "If you drop a frog in boiling water, it's going to scramble to get out, right?" Cecilia nods. "But if you put the frog in water and increase the temperature by increments, the frog will stay in the water. Eventually, the frog will boil." I look at her for a beat. "Benzos are the only drug that boil people. With long-term use, the brain loses its ability to regulate. Essentially, your brain is getting fried, but you don't realize it." I shift on the stool. It's so awkward, but I push forward. I pull out every analogy I can think of. I tell her benzodiazepines halt the body's ability to regulate brain traffic. "Imagine New York City with stuck traffic lights," I say. "It would be chaos, right? People are used to having a system tell them when to go and when to stop. So, with benzos, you have an outside force holding most of the lights on red. Only a few neurotransmitter cars get the green light. And if you think of New York City like a body, then no one is getting anywhere." Sweat beads on my forehead. I take a breath. "Does this make sense?"

"Absolutely," Cecilia says, nodding. "Go on."

"Okay, so if New York was a body and no cars or people were going anywhere, then parts of the city will start to die off. With benzos, your GABA receptors are the big regulators of neurotransmitter traffic. If no one gets through, the stomach can't digest food, the muscles don't know whether to contract or relax, the limbic/emotional system shuts down. I'm talking about over seventy percent of the body's functions being given a red light. Now, imagine that the outside force on the lights is pulled out. This is what happens when people reach tolerance or try to get off the benzos. The lights go all green and everything goes haywire."

I look over at Len. He's chewing his nails and staring into the little screen on the camera. He gives me a thumbs-up.

My legs stick together. I keep my back straight but not rigid. I try to relax. "Here's the thing that's the hardest to understand," I continue.

"The GABA receptors have gotten so used to being overruled by the benzos that they've actually stopped working. Some of them stop working for good, which is why it takes months and months for people to feel any semblance of normal. And, honestly, I wonder how fully the brain *can* recover. The pharmaceutical companies aren't going to look into that, I can promise you. And this is what scares me about benzos: people go under and they don't come back out for a long, long time. For me, it's been over a year and a half. It's terrifying."

Cecilia looks at me with sympathetic eyes. "So do you consider yourself fully recovered?"

I wonder how I can answer. Do I say that I consider myself lucky? Do I say that I've come to terms with the fact I may never sleep normally again—that I may always have a fragile nervous system?

"No," I say. "I'm not fully recovered. But I can walk. And I can eat. And I can hold my children. A year ago I couldn't have said that."

Len bends over and squints at one of the cameras. Two empty Diet Cokes have been kicked to the corner of the room. He stands and smiles. I feel like my heart might explode in my chest. God, I hope this makes sense. I hope I'm not babbling. *Keep going*, I think. *Say everything.*

"So here's the thing. Everyone agrees you shouldn't take benzos for more than four weeks at a time. Medical literature is very clear. But despite this, the medical establishment prescribes benzos like candy, all while refusing to do long-term studies. A lot of doctors don't know this." Cecilia raises her eyebrow. "It's true. Doctors are just as swayed by marketing as we are. We have evidence that benzos cause structural changes in the brain, but a lot of doctors have no idea. I know that researchers in the US and the UK have tried to put together studies, but no one will fund them. You can guess who shuts them down, right? What industry stands to lose great profit? So it boils down to this: we love our 'war on drugs' but the real back alley—the one we don't even know we're in—is our doctor's office."

"Cut!" Len yells from the kitchen. He's gone to get his third Diet Coke. He walks back into the living room. "Nice job," he says. "I think we've got it."

Len decides the last take will be the interview with Sean and me. We're told to stand near the kitchen table. It feels awkward, he says, but it won't look awkward. I know from watching news shows in the past that I should look at Sean when he's speaking. He talks, staring straight ahead. The tension feels tight enough to touch, a huge band pulled to the breaking point. Cecilia asks Sean what it was like watching me and he says it was like watching someone have their legs cut out from underneath them. I can't recall a time Sean has expressed awareness of how the withdrawal has impacted me, so his comment leaves me numb and confused. It all feels so staged, the milking of the emotion, the scripting of identity. Cecilia turns and says that she has just one last question for me.

"It's been said by many experts that benzo withdrawal is worse than getting off heroin. If this is the case, I want to know how you did it. You had two infants—one with Down syndrome. With all those factors stacked against you, how did you have the strength to get off? I just . . . I don't get it." And there's something about the way she asks that disarms me. She's not as poised and direct as she was with her other questions. She's softer, quieter.

"I'm not sure," I say. I stand for a beat, moving my palm over the top of the kitchen table. "I could tell you a thousand and one stories . . . but the truth is . . . I don't know . . ."

She shakes her head, uncomprehending.

"It's like when I was on the floor in Chloe's room. I was sure I was going to end up dead."

"But you didn't." Cecilia leans forward, imploring. "You didn't give up."

"No."

"You crawled. You kept going."

"Yeah." I look at her. "I wish I could tell you, but . . . something in me."

"You *wouldn't* give up."

"It wasn't even conscious . . . It's like when a bird learns to fly for the first time. There's no looking down to evaluate. That's not even an option. No matter how dark the night is or how far you might fall, you just do it. You find some way not to hit the ground."

# BENZOS DON'T
# HAVE CLEAVAGE

*February 2014*

TWO WEEKS LATER LEN TELLS ME to get the popcorn. It's happening. Sean says he doesn't want to watch the interview. His voice is cold and he doesn't offer an explanation. I don't argue. I'm at the point where I'd rather watch without him. I text Ann that she needs to be ready. The piece is going to air tonight. I text Ivy and Hollis and my mom. I email Matt. "This is it," I tell them. "We're going national." I tell them benzos will be the new black and they all laugh, and I feel so clever. I am up. I am euphoric this will be on prime time. Diane Sawyer cares and tonight she's going to make all of America care. News will erupt from the major networks. People will come out from the shadows. Prescribing policies will be reviewed and changed. There will be lawsuits and talk of requiring doctors to provide informed consent. There will be black box warnings with big letters and people will understand that with this family of drugs the brain can be permanently altered.

I'm feeling defiant. I'm feeling like a fucking champion. I've fought to make this story known. I've written innumerable blogs, pitched

*60 Minutes* and *Frontline* to deaf ears. But now, I have Diane Sawyer! I have prime time! People will know. People will be brought to their knees with the clear and unassailable truth.

Sean tells me not to get too excited. I've made celebratory lasagna and he says he'll watch the kids, but I shouldn't get my hopes up. I stare at him from across the table.

"What?" he asks.

"Don't get my hopes up?" I say. My voice has an edge.

"Yeah. Don't get your hopes up." He wipes Finch's face, which is decorated with tomato sauce.

"Thanks," I say. I step away from the edge. I don't want to sound angry. The kids are four and five now, so they get intonation. They get hostility that comes from a heart sinking just an inch or so lower in the chest. They may not understand what's going on, but they feel the force of it like a wind.

"I'm just happy something is going to be said," I add by way of recovery, "however small."

At 5:25 p.m., I go downstairs and turn on the television. Sean elects to stay upstairs with the kids. I bring my phone down because I know Ann is standing by.

*I have popcorn*, she texts.

*All engines a go*, I reply.

There's the grand swing of the camera toward Diane, starting high, then circling around to the back of the set and arriving dramatically as Diane looks up and into the camera. It's our eyes she's looking into. There's such intimacy, such purpose. And we're off. The first story is about a wildfire in Los Angeles. Oh, it's so fitting. *Wildfire*. I text Ann: *OMG. In California!* A massive blaze is threatening homes. And David Muir, the correspondent, is in the thick of it, reporting on the three degenerates who started the blaze with a careless campfire. We see mug shots, and all three are young and sour, with long, greasy hair. The correspondent looks grieved but stoic. He's wearing a yellow firefighter's jacket. His hair sits unmarred on his head, neatly shellacked against the heat.

*Nice hair*, Ann texts.

A minute later Diane shifts to a story about a twenty-two-year-old man who began shooting at an Elkhart, Indiana, supermarket. There are graphics to demonstrate the position of the shooter as he held the store manager hostage. There's another mug shot. We hear from the correspondent that, due to rapid response techniques, the police brought this young man down. The police look calm and determined. No time to wait for backup, the correspondent says. No time to wait for SWAT. The police must engage. They must *confront*.

Two minutes later, the next segment: contaminated water in West Virginia.

At 5:38 p.m., we hear the Senate has passed a compromise to avoid another government shutdown. At 5:39 p.m., Diane tells us of an urgent warning: hospital emergency room waits are long. It's awful. The nation's emergency care environment is at a breaking point. Don't go.

*Go only if you're not dying*, Ann texts.

*No, if you're dying, definitely go, but you might have to wait*, I respond.

Ann and I continue texting, joking about what's happening minute by minute in the show. It helps to have humor. It helps to have someone with me.

5:42 p.m.—the Australian Open was suspended due to heat. Something about an egg frying on the court.

5:43 p.m.—the number one fear in America is public speaking. There's a commercial break. A man punches out a life-size roasted chicken. Heartburn medication. Next, a lovely female doctor recommends a medicine for dry eye. It borders on tender, this dry eye issue.

We're back at 5:46 p.m. to explore the panic besetting most Americans, a fear more intense than the fear of dying.

Ann: *Hope you're not bumped . . . This is fluff!*

Another commercial break. More concern about the perils of heartburn. The purple pill can help. Side effects include bone fracture, headache, stomach pain, and persistent diarrhea. *Diarrhea*, I text. *Sexy.* Ah, another eye medicine. Car insurance. Aleve. Campbell's soup. The people in the commercials are friendly and approachable. Ann and I text on the merits of dating the actor in the Aleve commercial.

5:51 p.m.—Diane tells us it's time for the Instant Index. It's all going so fast. I can feel the clock ticking down. Pop icon Katy Perry lights up the screen. She's singing her hit single "Roar," which was nominated for song of the year in 2013. The set of the video is a jungle. Katy has been in a plane crash but has adapted well and even tamed a tiger.

Me: *Roar, Katy. Roar.*

Ann: *You can't be serious.*

Katy disappears and there is an ad for medication to help handsome men with their erectile dysfunction. Go to the emergency room if you experience an erection lasting more than four hours. Call your doctor if you have any decrease or loss in hearing or vision or if you can't breathe and your lips bleed. *Perhaps Katy can help them*, I think. *Perhaps she'll be my segue.*

Me: *No no!! Bumped and not even a call from the producer!*

Ann: *Not a text or email?*

Me: *No. He swore it would be on tonight.*

Ann: *I'm bummed. What should I do with all the popcorn?*

Minutes later, I get a text from Hollis: *Were you on? Did we miss you? Did they bump you for Katy Perry?*


I WATCH *ABC World News with Diane Sawyer* every night for the next week. I email Matt that I got bumped for Katy Perry. Len is frustrated but reassures me over the phone it *will* run. The networks always shuffle things. Stuff comes up. Some news has more urgency or is timelier. Take Vladimir Putin's homophobic comments at the Olympic Winter

Games. They had to run it. But then there's the piece on the best way to eat a hamburger to avoid burger slippage. This is news?

And then, on February 2, news breaks that Philip Seymour Hoffman has died of a drug overdose. This acting legend was found in his bathroom, needle still in his arm, glasses on his head. It's a blow. The networks go wild. There will be an autopsy, but the early belief is that Hoffman was "stacking." This is the term, we hear, for using multiple drugs, one on top of another. Networks hound Hoffman's friends and family. There are tearful comments that he died too soon, too young. We know this story. He struggled with addiction for so long. He was such a talent.

And I know this is it. This is the perfect segue. There were benzodiazepines in Hoffman's system. We know this.

I ask Sean if he wants to watch but, no, no, he doesn't want to. He will watch the kids again. "I'll give you that," he says.

At 5:36 p.m., the story starts. Chilling death scene. Needle in his arm. Seventy baggies of heroin. There are clips of Hoffman's performance as Truman Capote, the role that won him an Oscar. He was brilliant, the rare actor who could disappear into any role. And then the police scene. There are pictures of needles and I realize the focus is just on heroin. An expert comes on explaining about the euphoria that heroin produces, the high that we know and love to hear about. We see a hand holding a spoon with golden liquid. There's a lighter under the spoon—a needle hovering—

Jesus. We can't get enough of this image. We love it because we can hold the horror apart. *Not me. I'd never put a needle in my arm.*

There's no mention of the cocaine or amphetamines. No mention of benzodiazepines. They're going to skip it. They're exploiting the well-played heroin horror story: the needle in the arm, death in the bathroom, lights on Broadway dimmed. His poor family, Diane says. This drug has torn them apart. They don't run my story. Instead, Cecilia Vega is interviewed. She's with Diane and her soft eyes. Cecilia's dad was a heroin addict. He overdosed when she was little. "He just couldn't do it," Cecilia says, her voice soft. "He chose heroin over life." Goddamn it, ABC. *Benzodiazepines* ruin families. They ruin *lives*. But benzodiazepines don't have the dirty glamour of heroin. No track marks or back alleys with benzos. The horrors of benzos exist in their perfect legality, in the lackluster regulation and the culture that treats them like cocktail party candies. People may be able to push heroin into a narrative they feel safe from, but benzos are much closer to home. When we feel sick or sleepless or crushed by life, we listen to our doctor. I know this. But still. *Still, Diane*. You chose the easy heroin seduction over the lurking shadow in our doctors' offices, the one just as damaging as heroin. Goddamn.

Len stops calling me after the first week. Two months later I call ABC about the piece. I'd love a copy of the footage, I say. It wasn't run but it means something to me. I'm told that Len is no longer working with ABC and that producers typically take the footage if it isn't aired. I look Len up on LinkedIn a year later and discover that he's taken a job with a pharmaceutical company. The piece wasn't run, he likely has the footage, and now he's working for Big Pharma. It's like a bad movie with me as the walk-on.

# THE BOOK OF WAKING

*March 2014*

AFTER ABC, IT DOESN'T TAKE LONG for the spiral down between
Sean and me to reach the end. ABC provided a brief period of denial,
a time when hope rode high over the black cloud in our house. But
once the surge of distraction ends, we break ourselves against the constant arguments. We argue over the pieces of dental floss Sean leaves
on the counter. We argue about the cheese and bread moldering in the
fridge. We argue over the dishes and the lasagna and the empty sky.
We argue as if fighting will erase the anguish between us, but nothing
gives. There are not enough mountains for Sean to hike, and I feel
his constant need to be away, to be anywhere but here, like a bruise.
There's no blame in this. I could no more have expected Sean to stand
next to me in my pain unmarked than I could have expected water not
to be wet.

And this is the truth of things. The knowing comes to me like
a seed bursting open. Resentment and grief have grown mountains
inside us, and we can't seem to get to their summit. We can't conquer
them. The stakes of pain have been high enough for me to finally let
go. So I do.

Sean has come in from outside. I'm sitting at the kitchen table. Chloe and Finch are asleep and the house has a humming quiet. Sean walks in and grabs a glass for water. He leans against the sink, glass aloft, staring past me into the vacant living room. In that moment I know. We turned away from each other long ago and our pain has grown pale and sick in that turning. We failed each other but, really, who's to say? Relationships die for lesser things. We have nothing left for each other, and sitting there, watching his eyes far from here, I know I'll break from this broken marriage. Sean will climb his mountains to sit and cry and I will not stay with him. There's a new tenderness in my body, a sprout gingerly rising out of the soil. I want to protect and nourish this sprout. I want to take this new health and love in my body and nourish it in sunlight.

I run my hand over the kitchen table, my finger tracing the scratches, feeling the slight hollow running a line under my skin. Sean's body is stiff, held away from me by a pain that seems to extend beyond his body, past the house and trees and sky. "I want a separation," I say. "We've been through so much." Sean stares at the wall behind me and I wait, fingering the wood, watching the bony trees outside the window. He pauses, then says I'm either in or out. There will be no in between. And that's it. It's over.

Sean takes two weekends to move out. He packs up the office and the kitchen and the bathroom. We go through the house and decide who gets the couch, the refrigerator, the big mirror over the bed. Who gets the panini press I picked out as a wedding gift, the Crate and Barrel plates? A week later Sean takes Finch and Chloe to visit his mother in Idaho. Sharon tells him he can't get divorced. She tries every angle to convince him and lands on the fact that, if nothing else, he should stay with me for the sex. When he gets back, we laugh at that one. Oh, it's good. We laugh together even as we hurt each other in a million other ways, even as we split up the knives.

After Sean leaves, I begin listening to a lot of music. Our house has been absent of music. I didn't realize but we don't even have a radio. I put my computer on the couch in the living room and find the recording of Adele doing a tiny desk concert at NPR. Jesus, that voice. I stare at my computer screen, tears streaming down my face. Adele with her long lashes and her rolling-in-the-deep voice. Finch and Chloe color on big stacks of paper on the floor, and I help Chloe with her little bird picture, the big-eyed bird inside an awkward egg.

And then, as the weeks go on, there's so much music. Sean and I agree on joint custody and we tell Finch and Chloe they'll have two homes and a mama and papa who adore them. And it's here, in the space of my aloneness, that I come back to myself. I'm no longer sick. I'm no longer disabled by drugs or loss. My body fills with music and I keep listening; my body is a joyful beatbox, a harp, a piano trill. Somewhere in those years of being sick and lost in the dark, I found an unknown light within me. I found my way out of the dark with that light. I won't get lost again.

There are musicians I know and musicians I don't know who have recorded their songs at a little NPR desk—the books stacked floor to ceiling—the feel at once bohemian and professional and urgent. I watch these musicians sing in a space the size of a bathroom, the size of a desk, and they have so much energy, so much life, I cry and keep crying at the beauty, the tiny beauty of it all.

Chloe loves watching the desk concerts on the computer, so we make our way through them all. I tell Finch and Chloe about the blues and beatboxing, about hip-hop and flamenco and punk anthems and disco. My God, I say, who is this Macklemore jumping like a pogo stick? Who is this other guy who makes music with plastic bottles and sings about water birds? Mostly I listen and cry. I help color Chloe's birds orange and blue and fuchsia. I don't make clouds. We listen to the Preservation Hall Jazz Band, and the raw energy of those instruments makes the air in the living room vibrate. Finch wants me to draw a hippo. He wants to draw pictures of flowers and butterflies and pictures of a home that still have Daddy in them.

At night I cook Moroccan chicken or burgers and we listen to ABBA, the Bee Gees, and Peaches & Herb. Chloe gains an appreciation for the songs "Brick House" and her all-time favorite "Shake Your Groove Thing." I start teaching the two of them how to shake it in the kitchen. We eat and then Chloe will say, "Groovy song, Mama," and I put the song on, and we wiggle all over that white tile. We shake it in front of the bay window looking out to the street. We shake it down the hall and back and I explain the art of the disco turn to Finch: Right foot out and spin on your toe to face the direction you just came from, pointer fingers like guns at the ready.

"Get your pointer fingers up," I yell at Finch as he wiggles down the hallway, forgetting his spin and walking instead into the bathroom.

"One, two, three, turn!" I say to Chloe as she spins and spins, getting dizzy, the smile on her face big as a comet.

And sometimes I start crying again, but I'm laughing too. I spin with my pointers and pick up Finch and swing him around that big kitchen. Then Chloe lifts her arms to be picked up, so I play the song again and spin her and her giggle is like spring—it's like something new growing inside me. "Hands on your hips, Finch," I yell, moving my hips back and forth to show him. Chloe runs over and mimics me. We name our dances—the butter churn, the washing machine, the milkshake. These are our days and our nights. We dance and listen to music. We sit on the porch, watching the sky, and we color the windows green and orange and electric blue. *I will make a new home*, I think. *I will make a new place for us to live. I have crawled out of an underworld of near death and all I see now is life. I will help all of us grow and unfurl until our little sprout bodies lift up out of the soil, until we burst into the sun.*

# METAPHOR OF THE HOLES

*October 2015*

It's 2015. The Year of the Goat. The year of pitching over sideways and jumping up grinning. It's the year of the holes and hallelujah.

Finch, Chloe, and I have been living in the butter and lilac room at Hollis and Jerome's for a year and a half. We moved in just after Sean and I sold our house. My health is still fragile and I'm unemployed and they've taken us in. We eat dinners together at the big table under the Chihuly glass chandelier. The kids watch deer run through the backyard. Sean and I decide on a fifty-fifty coparenting agreement. We're cordial and keep our focus on the kids, though he often erupts with rage and resentments, which I feel powerless to address. Just months after we move in, I decide to run a Kickstarter to fund the first stage of writing this book. I didn't write at all through 2013 and wrote very little in 2014. I was too sick. But now I feel a garden of creativity in me. I'm a million little seeds bursting open. I hire a film crew. We make a beautiful video for the Kickstarter. I contact everyone I know. The Kickstarter funds in three days, so I have the equivalent of minimum wage for eight months. This is enough. This is more than I could have dreamed. I get the first draft out. I edit two or three times, all the while sending out résumés because I have no idea what I'll do for work. Just as the money is running out, I get a call from a friend. She knows of a job in IT, and it's crazy, but they just might hire me. After an interview—during which I'm asked questions saturated with acronyms I don't understand and after which I'm sure they'll cough loudly and hang up the phone—I have a job.

One month later, with the kids at Sean's, I get up to make coffee. The coffee press sits next to the sink and I've filled it with grounds and hot water. I'm holding the press with my left hand when I see the press moving in my peripheral vision. My arm, which does not feel like an arm, drifts across the ruby-colored tile, French press in hand. It's graceful and slow as spilling water and it doesn't feel like my arm. I grab it with my right. I make the fingers, which don't feel like fingers, let go of the handle. I watch my arm float like so much seaweed in a gentle ocean.

I decide, as all very stupid people decide, that this is no big deal. I feel disoriented, but I can walk a straight line and I'm sure if I tried to talk there'd be no problem. I sit on the couch and have a heart-to-heart with the powers that be. *Just in case this is something, I want you to know that I'm not ready. I want to see my kids grow up and I want to see this book published and I just got a job. So if it really is my time, I obviously can't argue, but I'm not giving the go-ahead. I'd rather stay for a while longer if you don't mind.*

After an hour I knock on Hollis's door. I didn't want to wake her up.

"Hollis," I whisper. "I think I might need an aspirin."

Two days later my vision gets wavy. I text Dr. Kate and she tells me to go to the emergency room *now*. It feels silly, but I drive myself down and shuffle to the front desk. Glass pane window, blond nurse inside with monitors in front of her, no one waiting.

"Yes?"

"Hey there. Um . . . I might be having a stroke. Or a TIA—one of those smaller strokes. I can't be sure." I'm casual, leaning against the thin counter. "It's probably nothing, but my doctor wanted me to come."

When I'm led to the antiseptic glow of the curtained room, I joke with the handsome male nurse. I ask about the craziest thing he's seen in the ER and he's clearly had this request before. He tells me, "Pool balls in the rectum. Some guy. You know." He raises his eyebrows.

"No!" I say, laughing like I'm at a big bar, instead of in a room with scrubbed tile and invasive digital machines. "Oh, that's just . . . Wow."

"Yeah," he says, plugging the heart monitor in. "He had to go into surgery. Poor guy had to call his mom."

I'm seen by the doctor on call, who advises an MRI. I'm still joking an hour later when the same male nurse comes back to tell me I'm staying. They're taking me upstairs. I've had an acute ischemic attack in the front parietal section of my brain. Stroke. And not just one, I'm told. There are two distinct white spots in my brain—two definitive strokes—one of which is older than the one I've come in for. After reviewing, Dr. Kate determines it was very likely the time I fell in Chloe's room. The time I crawled up the stairs and to the bedroom, unable to stand or talk. There's been no other incident so consistent with stroke symptoms.

"You're lucky you're still talking," the nurse says.

The stroke unit is on the fifth floor. Every vital sign is monitored. I'm hooked in with tubes and wires and they start me on blood thinners. The on-call neurologist visits. He seems to like me because of my history of insomnia. I'm a case that's interesting, because I don't fit the profile of a stroke victim. They need to find out why I've stroked out so they can prevent it from happening again.

Four days later, after innumerable tests, X-rays, and CAT scans, they find it. I have two holes in my heart. Patent foramen ovales, also called PFOs, are unremarkable. During fetal development, a small flap-like opening—the foramen ovale—is normally present in the wall between the right and left upper chambers of the heart. This hole normally closes after birth but about 25 percent of the population is walking around with PFOs of varying degrees. The big ones are the ones that cause problems. And they find out I don't just have one biggie. I have two. Two biggies and a blood clot that would normally be filtered through the lungs and *wham*—blood clot to the brain. Stroke.

I have two cardiologists. One is from Ghana and talks to me for half an hour about how people need to read more. I love this man. The other is the surgeon. I'm told on day five they need to close the holes. They'll insert a tiny Gore-Tex patch into my femoral artery and guide it up to my heart, where it will spread open like a slim Chinese lantern. Cells will cover it and my heart will effectively be spackled and patched up.

My room is filled with flowers. Ivy comes and opens a paper bag of rose petals that drift onto my thin white blanket. I'd called Sean when I was in the emergency room to tell him he'd need to keep the kids until the doctors figured out what was happening. He was toneless and focused on logistics, which made things easier. Our relationship, even with me in the hospital, is walled off from any emotion or warmth. He calls the day before my heart surgery and I break for the first time, crying over the phone. I'm worried that if the surgery doesn't go well, I won't be around for the kids. Sean offers what he can. "Do you want me to bring the kids tonight?" I do and he does and while he's stiff, the kids and I play on the bed that lifts up and down at the push of a button. We shuffle down the hall and I let Chloe push my IV pole while Finch says hello to all the nurses. I tell Chloe the doctors will fix my heart and I'll be home in no time. By the end of their visit, I feel strong. I burn for this living that's been given to me. Being mama to Finch and Chloe is a gift I refuse to give up.

"You okay?" my friends ask. "This must be so scary."

After one and a half years of detoxing off benzos, a stroke and heart surgery feel like a piece of cake. I have a posse of doctors and nurses caring for me. Friends and family call at all hours offering support. We understand what's happening and we know how to solve it. There are tests we can point to and say, *There, that's the offending clot. Those are the unfortunate holes.* There's a recovery plan and there's little pain. No part of me feels afraid, although I have no guarantee I'll make it out of surgery unscathed. Instead, I feel lucky. Making it through benzo detox was a brutal physical, emotional, spiritual boot camp, with no guarantee I'd ever get out. But I got out. And now I feel like a fucking gladiator.

During my time in the hospital, I walk around the stroke unit and talk with all those who can talk. I sit with them and listen to their stories. A woman just east of my room cries out for help at night because of an infection in her brain, and I hold her hand as often as the nurses let me. I am lucky. Aftereffects of the stroke show up only as a slight slowness on my left side. No biggie. I'll be racing up mountains before they know it.

And the metaphor of the holes provides the kind of poetic ending I couldn't have imagined. My heart had holes. I walked around with them my entire life, feeling lost and scared and wounded. But now I'm patched. After years in the arena, I've built muscle. After raging at the doors of death, all I care about now is living fully. Fear has been burned out of me.

# AFTER

*December 2021*

IN 2012, WHEN I was writing all the blogs for Mad in America chronicling my attempts to get off benzodiazepines, I received hundreds of emails from people. Some were fellow sufferers desperate to get off them and begging for advice on how to do so successfully. Some of the emails were from parents or siblings of people who had struggled with benzodiazepine dependence and lost. While each message was heartfelt and often full of anguish specific to their experience, what they shared was the question of whether I'd made it. As one would ask a veteran of an unnamed war, they wanted to know not just how I'd fought the battle but whether I'd survived. And to each one I said an unequivocal "*Yes.*"

It's now over a decade since my first prescription for Ativan and over five years since I've been at an amount of Valium my doctors feel will not cause further decline. The perfect conclusion to this story would be that I got off benzodiazepines entirely. That would be the bright and shiny Hollywood version, with me rising up with wings, triumphant and without a trace of the medication that nearly took my life. But this isn't the case. I dropped nearly to point zero, but divorce, being a mother to two, and facing the need to provide for my children made the final drop untenable. I still take 5 milligrams of Valium nightly. I hope to get off it someday, but for now, I accept that my brain is different from how it was before I began taking these drugs. I accept the vulnerability I feel every time I refill my prescription. And the truth is, with my health once again vibrant, the thought of going into the darkness of withdrawal is a terror I don't want to face. I live with an imperfect ending that humbles and emboldens me. I will never take my health for granted and I will always work to advocate for those suffering from benzodiazepine dependence.

So this is my *yes*. My children are eleven and twelve now and I support them by working a full-time job, and in the in-between hours I write. This alone is something I couldn't have imagined five years ago. I practice yoga in our living room and teach my children headstands. We make up plays in the dark with my serving as director and lighting designer with a series of flashlights. I am, in this moment, working to teach Finch how to tie his shoes. I should make mention at this point that Finch is not his real name. I have changed a few names in the book, my children's included. Beyond that, everything in this book is true and in keeping with my memory of the events, much of that memory pulled from the journals and blogs I kept through the whole experience.

At this writing, we are ten months into the Covid-19 pandemic and I'm acutely aware that prescription and use of benzodiazepines are skyrocketing. Many celebrities are coming out as having addictions to Xanax and many more who came before them have died as a result of their use. In an interview with Katie Couric, musician Chance the Rapper said he used to be addicted to Xanax. In 2015, he claimed that "Xanax is the new heroin." And in a 2019 *Vogue* article, Justin Bieber admitted to suffering a Xanax addiction, noting that "it got pretty dark. I think there were times when my security was coming in late at night to check my pulse and see if I was still breathing." No surprise. When Soundgarden lead singer Chris Cornell's death was ruled a suicide, his wife took the doctor who gave Chris innumerable prescriptions for Ativan to court.

She publicly blamed the Ativan the doctor had prescribed for her husband's death. The song "Black Hole Sun" rings hollow in the wake of Cornell's death. It's the perfect image for Ativan—a drug that promises light and then crushes the life out of you.

In late September 2020, the FDA issued a report that benzodiazepines would now be required to have stronger warning labels. The agency found that the current labeling information on the drugs "does not provide adequate warnings about the serious risks and harms associated with these medicines," adding that addiction could happen in a matter of days. One month later the government of Canada issued a similar report. In the first year of my withdrawal, I reported Dr. Amazing to the only state agency having a criminal unit for investigation into physician malpractice. A narcotics agent interviewed me and called both Dr. James and Dr. Kate just once, leaving messages. He spoke to neither of them, despite their calls back to him, and the case was quietly closed. Dr. Amazing remains in practice to this day.

# NEVER NOT BROKEN

*January 2023*

It's been more than twelve years since Dr. Amazing gave me my first prescription for benzodiazepines. People have asked me over the years if I've ever gone back to see him. "Does he know?" they've asked. "Could you face him?" "No," I'd told the mom of a daughter in Chloe's class, "I haven't given him my book. I have no desire to confront him. He's just one doctor. There are thousands." Until recently, I hadn't been able to imagine facing the man whose medical decisions delivered years of quiet violence, years of anguish. What would I say? Would I swing a bat? Would I unleash on him about the collective hubris and neglect of the medical establishment? Would I force a bolus of words down his throat like that of a goose whose liver I'd later pull out, grind up, and mash onto fancy crackers at a dinner party? Would I make him choke?

While researching this book, I called his office to get my medical records. *Yes, I could get a copy of my records*, the receptionist said with a lifted and reassuring voice. She'd have them at the front desk. Dr. Amazing was not in town; I made sure I didn't go there when he was. The thought of walking in and talking to the man whose prescriptions had taken me to the brink of death and disability was like asking someone to throw a baseball *hard* at the center of my chest.

But this was only partly true.

The other truth lives in a place in me I've wanted to keep hidden, the part that feels always and forever broken. This part moves through the world, still shattered at the dismissal of the benzo epidemic. The thought of facing Dr. Amazing was like inviting the deadly indifference of the world. Much of the medical community still denies the savagery benzos can wreak on the brain. *It can't be that bad*, goes the rhetoric. *I've never had a patient complain.* Shame festers in invisibility, and invisibility persists when scientific truths are eclipsed by a whitewash of marketing prowess. According to J. C. Ballenger in a 1988 article published in *Archives of General Psychiatry*,\* the makers of Xanax cited statistics from only week four of a fourteen-week study of the drug to claim efficacy against placebo in managing panic disorder. At four weeks, Xanax showed improvement over placebo for the study participants. However, at the end of eight weeks (active treatment phase), there was no statistically significant difference on most of the rating scales, at least among those who remained in the study. What the investigators didn't show is that at eight weeks, those on Xanax began a six-week taper to get off the drug. At the end of the taper, 39 percent of the study participants had deteriorated to such a degree that they had to resume taking the benzodiazepine, 35 percent suffered rebound panic and anxiety symptoms more severe than when the study began, and 35 percent suffered distressing symptoms they had never experienced before. In sum, at the end of the full fourteen-week study, those who had taken Xanax actually were more phobic, were more anxious, suffered more panic attacks, and were doing worse on a global scale

---

\* J. C. Ballenger et al., "Alprazolam in panic disorder and agoraphobia: results from a multicenter trial. I. Efficacy in short-term treatment." *Arch Gen Psychiatry* 45, no. 5 (May 1988): 413–22, doi: 10.1001/archpsyc.1988.01800290027004.

that's designed to assess overall well-being. This manipulation of the clinical trials and the misrepresentation of findings skew greatly in the manufacturer's favor. Add to this the vigorous marketing of Xanax for panic disorder and you have a drug being proffered as a balm for a chronic condition when its own trials showed that its efficacy soured and it even made participants increasingly more anxious and sleepless after a month. But when the marketing took off, benzos once again became a long-term cultural salve. This deliberate calculation of profit over patient health and safety stole my breath for years.

*Blood Orange Night* was first published in June 2022. I've done innumerable interviews and podcasts since then, and interviewers often ask me whether I consider myself an addict. This is a fair question and one I've wrestled with for years. Was I? What did that even mean, to be an addict? I finally landed on the fact that our cultural narrative of addiction makes us "other" addicts to such a degree that we feel safe in our distance from them. We feel that we do not have to see them as human beings just like us, people with the same human needs, desires, and sources of suffering that we all experience. Essentially, *they* are not *us*. The word itself has tremendous weight. Addicts, the cultural narrative goes, are bad. They're unhinged, running around with a broken moral compass, with shame as their legacy. We in the benzo community don't want to be lumped in with the "addicts." We don't want to be *them*, the broken ones. Most of us received a prescription from a doctor to remedy some form of suffering and we followed our doctor's orders. We became "physically dependent," but we hadn't "used." We weren't off the rails; we weren't just looking for a high. But this is a limited perspective. As humans, we all experience suffering, and we all search for a means by which we can alleviate our suffering. Shame shouldn't exist in this equation, and the language of addiction is the language of shame. I was, in part, afraid to bring my book into the world and into Dr. Amazing's office because I still felt the resin of shame. I wanted to walk through the world fearless and unapologetic, but a small, hidden part of me still felt broken, embarrassed, and filled with shame. Maybe I simply hadn't been strong enough. Maybe some *weakness*, a dark shadow in me, had fallen prey to the drugs. I feared the pointed fingers—I feared dismissal—I feared my own fragility.

When I was a wild and naive eighteen-year-old, I traveled to Nepal and discovered a love of Eastern spiritual practices. I learned yoga and meditation in Kathmandu. I trekked to that country's Solu Khumbu region and sat cross-legged with enlightened masters. I took their teachings and tried to meditate away the pain of my childhood. It helped, but the dark seed of sadness stayed in me. *Maybe it will never go away*, I thought. *Maybe I'll always be just a little bit broken.*

And when I fell into benzo dependency and the time of true darkness came, everything I thought I'd come to understand about myself and the world around me unraveled. I fell so far, so fast, there was not enough left to even hold the sense of being broken. I was that child flung from a spinning merry-go-round, and I hit the ground so hard, all my breath shot out of me.

I lay on that metaphorical ground, aching to breathe, for years.

In writing everything down for this book, I finally saw myself. I cut myself open and bled my brokenness onto the page. I let myself see everything in me that made me feel as if I couldn't go on and watched the part of me that stood up anyway. There was no hiding.

In Hindu mythology there is a goddess whose name translates as *Never Not Broken*. When I heard of Akhilandeshvari, the forever broken goddess who rides on the back of a crocodile, I realized I'd found my muse. This goddess teaches that we derive our power from being broken, from living in flux and constantly emerging into different selves that, by their very nature, are limitless. Instead of existing as a fixed identity, the Never Not Broken goddess rides a crocodile in a state that's constantly *becoming*. Like a multifaceted prism with color shooting out from our crystalline cuts, it's in our fractures that we reveal our full beauty.

I called Dr. Amazing's office six months after my book was published. *Could I bring Dr. Amazing a gift?* I asked the receptionist. *Could I drop by after his last patient of the day so that I could deliver it personally?* Her response was sharp and cool. *I could drop by as long as I was brief. Dr. Amazing finished at 3:30 and would be out the door at 3:45*, she told me. I had my window.

The clinic had moved locations since I'd been there, more than a decade ago. It was now a few miles away, on the bottom floor of a featureless two-story office building that could as easily have housed an accounting or insurance firm. I sat in the car for a full five minutes, feeling my heart thump a hot fist against my chest. I had no idea what to expect.

The office was quiet, with bright fluorescent lights and gray carpeting that was both utilitarian and cold. The large front room faced the check-in window, with back offices to the right and a large square waiting room to the left. A narrow hallway cut through the middle and led, I could only guess, to Dr. Amazing's office. The waiting room was empty except for four metal chairs set at precise right angles to one another around an even smaller square table. A single wall facing the table and chairs had been painted an emphatic purple.

I checked in with the woman at the front desk. *Yes, I could wait*, she told me, reminding me that Dr. Amazing was busy. She looked down at the yellow gift bag with orange tissue paper in my hand. "I'll let him know you're here," she said, and nodded to the waiting area.

I sat in the chair that would give me the best view of the hallway to the back offices. I checked my watch—3:10 in the afternoon.

I waited.

3:30. The purple wall was really loud.

No one came in or out. The hum of fluorescent lights pulsed. The glare of winter gray from the big window looking out onto the street leaked into the room. I waited.

At 3:45 a door shut. I heard a shuffle on the utilitarian carpet, and then he was in front of me, his smile bright as a Florida sun.

I don't remember exactly what he said. He beamed, welcoming. I told him I'd brought a gift. *Did he know I'd written a book?* "No," he said, leaning back slightly. "I had no idea." I pulled the book out of the bag, a lit torch. "Here," I said. "I'd love for you to read it."

He held it to his chest and thanked me. I asked whether he had a few moments to talk, but he gestured to the hallway and said he had a patient waiting. He was late. He must get to them. "Will you call me once you've read the book?" I asked. "I'd love to talk with you about it." He agreed. He seemed genuine, but I didn't quite believe him.

"I'm going on a trip in a few days," he said. "I'll read it while I'm out of town."

I thought that would be the end.

I thought he'd place the book on a table somewhere far from here and walk away, but he didn't. He called twice just before the Christmas holiday. "Call me," he said. "I'm nearly done with the book."

We texted a few times and agreed to meet at the Tea Grotto, a fancy teahouse in Salt Lake, once he was back from his trip. We met there on January 7. It was early evening and the warm, amber lighting in the Grotto softened my nerves. As I got out of my car, I saw Dr. Amazing through the glass windows. He was standing near the long marble countertop that separated the main room from the wall that featured dozens of herbal and wellness teas. He wore an elegant coat that dropped to his ankles. He fidgeted with something in his hands and looked around. He was stiff when I walked in. We stood back from each other, awkward with the weight of the unsaid. We walked to the counter to order, awkward in the pretense we were just two friends getting together on a cold day in a warm teahouse, nothing more. He bought me green tea with roasted rice. Somehow, the cherished private alcove in the back corner of the front room was empty. It was as if the world had opened up a small chapel for us to talk.

I'd spent the entire holiday and the days leading up to our meeting thinking about what I would say to him. Did I want him to understand what I'd gone through? Did I want him to feel the burn of shame? Did *I* want to be the one to cast that scalding coal of shame into his house?

*Never Not Broken*, I thought. What would it be to sit with him and quietly listen to what he had to say? What would it be to walk in without trying to pull myself together and to believe that he might also carry within him a place that was broken? What would it be to sit in the space of our shared humanity? I knew that to walk in rigid in my beliefs about him would not let any light in. I had to shake myself out. I had to go into that little teahouse chapel and sit in the space of vulnerability.

He talked for an hour, his voice sounding at once anxious and intelligent. He was, I imagined, used to talking, used to being listened to. But this was different. He was facing someone whose life had come crashing down as a result of his prescribing. He had no clue what I wanted from him.

He sat to my right, staring ahead, his hands repeatedly lifting up from his lap like tired birds and smacking against the teak table in front of us. Back in New York, when he'd just begun his practice, he told me, there'd been a time when things were falling apart. The birds lifted and dropped, hitting the teak table with an erratic rhythm. He'd gone through a period of two weeks when he didn't sleep. "I remember thinking, 'If anyone tells me to take a hot bath again, I'm going to pummel them,'" he said. He sat at the edge of the wooden bench in our tea chapel, his back almost painfully straight. He looked over at me briefly. Benzos had been his savior back then. He'd used them off and on for years and never had a problem, never had more than a few nights of interrupted sleep. He was sorry, he said, his voice at such a steady run there was no room for conversation unless I talked over him. He remembered my level of desperation when I'd come to see him. I'd gone to everyone under the sun—naturopaths, general practitioners, therapists, shamans—he remembered that. He'd only wanted to help.

I sat in the space of that little chapel and looked at the small chip on the teacup, the lines carved into the wood table, the tired bird hands in Dr. Amazing's lap. We are all Never Not Broken. My body felt loose and hot. I made a few comments here and there, but I'd said what I had to say in the book. It was his turn. He told me that all he'd learned about benzos in medical school was that they were better than barbiturates and not addictive. This was a long time ago, back when benzos were new and the horror stories of dependence and withdrawal hadn't yet emerged. Like me, he'd believed what he was told. I glanced at him—the man who had been willing to meet me after reading my book—and I understood. He'd been broken back in New York, his medical training had not alerted him to the dangers of benzos, and he had wanted to help. That was all. Maybe he should have been more attentive. Maybe he should have been more up to date on the medical literature. Maybe he should have checked in, but the truth was, his suffering was my suffering. He'd wanted to help, and nothing in his experience had given him the eyes my book had given him.

We talked about what he'd seen in his practice over the past several years. The stress of a worldwide pandemic, political chaos, financial instability, inflation, and war abroad had created an epidemic of overwhelm. "Everyone that comes in," he said, "is just fried beyond belief." I nodded. The world at large felt fractured, unstable, and in flux.

We finished our tea. Dr. Amazing stood up and put on his long coat. We walked outside, into the light sleet falling from an indigo sky.

"Thank you for making time to talk," I said.

He stood in front of the glass door to the Tea Grotto. Car lights hitting the drizzle of rain and snow turned the drops into tiny fireflies. He nodded. "I've learned a lot that's very important," he said, looking up into the wet sky. "From your book."

*That's everything I could have hoped for*, I thought. I walked back to my car, watching the fireflies of the night. *Thank you*, I whispered to the universe, my heart radiating with the light of a forgiveness I hadn't even realized I needed.

# ACKNOWLEDGMENTS

THERE IS NO sufficient way to say, "Thank you for my life," but I shall endeavor. To Dr. Kate and Dr. James, you gave me hope and held me up when I was sure I wasn't likely meant for this earth. May your patients know how damn lucky they are to have you.

Brent Ottley and Chris Rogers, there's no way to express how your calm abiding and crazy needle ninja skills kept me together. Thank you to everyone who works at Wasatch Community Acupuncture for providing low-cost acupuncture, so I could rebuild my nervous system. Your nonprofit clinic is a vision of solid social justice work in health care. Thank you also to People's Organization of Community Acupuncture (POCA) for building the model of affordable and accessible acupuncture to reduce individual and collective suffering. I don't know if I would have made it without you.

Gerald and Elise Lazar, you were both nest and heartbeat for me when God knows I needed both. Your warmth and generosity are big enough to light a city. You brought together the Imagine Dream Team and mercy; the joy is a running river. Hilary, Neva, Janice, Sander, Jed, Sophia, Sage, Jessica, and the next mystery guest: how I love you all.

Finch and Chloe, you may never know what you mean to me. I only want you to fly with great joy lighting your wings. Watching you grow those wings blows my mind daily. I adore you with every fiber of my being.

To the staff at the Mount Olympus Presbyterian Church childcare center. Thank you for doing everything you could to care for Finch. You gave me a tremendous head start and I'll be forever grateful for your enduring kindness to me and my family.

Mom, thank you for standing next to me and holding my hand for so many months. You understood my pain and that was everything. Dad and Chris—thank you for supporting me in every way you could. It must have been terrifying to watch from afar and have no idea what was happening to me.

A huge and messy hug to both Matt Samet and Robert Whitaker. You were my lanterns in the dark when I was reaching out of the crevasse of benzo dependence. I called you my heroes back then and you remain so to this day. What luck to have found you.

Thank you to the writing group I've been in longer than my marriage: Dorothee Kocks, Brenda Sue Cowley, Kevin Jones, Stephen Trimble, Dave Jones, and Kurt Proctor. You saw me at my messiest and most desperate and still you saw the light of the poet. You are a joy of a writing family and the thrum of our meetings and weekends gave me enough reminders of what I loved to keep me stitched together. We're a motley, lively, hot toddy of a crew and I couldn't have kept at this without you.

My deepest thanks and most sincere apologies to the readers of my massive and untamed 450-plus-page vomitorium of a first draft—Jonathan, Sheryl, Lisa, Beth, and anyone else who was daring or foolish enough to read it. You dove in to being my first beta readers and for this I'll be forever grateful.

To Ann, without whom I wouldn't have survived the summer of 2011. You are sunshine and discoverer of the elusive mouth unicorn. I am forever grateful.

To Jeremy, who is undiluted love and who taught me it's not the knock down; it's the get up. Believe it, baby.

Mark Malatesta, you gave me the machete to find the trail to publishing. Your honesty, integrity, and belief in me were everything.

My agent, Jen Nadol—who knew I'd find the one and perfect person for me? The fact that you live in an old barn is what drew me in (the romanticism of such a thing!); your brilliance and solid, guiding hand gave my wild energy a place to flow. And Rebecca Strobel—who knew I could find an editor on whom I'd also have a girl crush? You saw all the places I held back and helped me to be more honest. You were those X-ray eyes I needed. You even watched my Instagram videos, the ones I sent with my hallmark giddy enthusiasm, and never once coughed and asked to please be excused. We are *on* that roller-coaster ride and I promise I'll keep bringing the popcorn.

Sara, Amie, Pam, Kindra, Ben, Sander, Jed, Sage, G-love—thanks for the nuggets of joy you gave when you could.

Peter Yarrow—you'll never know the simple kindness you offered and how much strength it gave me.

This would not be complete if I didn't give a shout-out to my Kickstarter supporters—THOSE TO WHOM I OWE EVERYTHING. There were nearly a hundred of you who believed enough that I could write this book that you put up cold hard cash. You should know you kept me and the kids afloat in 2015. Your collective support was a buoy I held on to while writing the first draft of *Blood Orange Night*. Thank you with all my heart for trusting me and believing I could do it. (Leslie and Lee—I still owe you. Let me buy you both a cup of tea.)

And a lifetime of thanks to the late Professor Heather Ashton for her legacy of over thirty years of benzodiazepine research. Her devotion to the people suffering benzodiazepine dependence and withdrawals gave many of us a chance at survival. She is deeply missed.

# ABOUT THE AUTHOR

**Melissa Bond** began the first poetry slam in Salt Lake City in 1996 at the Lazy Moon Pub. She ran it single-handedly for eight years, at which point it had strong enough legs to continue on its own. She started honing her skills as a narrative journalist in the 1990s and wrote for nearly every periodical in Salt Lake City. She was later an associate editor and poetry editor of the *Wasatch Journal*, a glossy long-form magazine serving the Intermountain West. In the years of her dependence on benzodiazepines, Melissa began her own blog and became a regular contributor to Mad in America. The University of Utah Medical School profiled her in a short film in 2017, and she was invited to give a talk at the University of Utah's medical anthropology department. *ABC World News with Diane Sawyer* contacted her for an interview, which was filmed in January 2014. Melissa is a respected writer on the perils of overprescribing benzodiazepines and is regularly featured in the online platforms Mad in America, Ravishly, and Catalyst. She has been featured on the podcasts *Risk!*, *IGNTD*, and *The Addiction Podcast*. She is scheduled as a keynote speaker at the National Coalition Against Prescription Drug Abuse conference in 2022 and was a guest speaker at the National Association for Down Syndrome in 2021. She lives in Utah with her two children, one of whom was the inspiration behind her short film, *Gooogled*, which premiered at the San Jose International Short Film Festival. To find out more, visit www.MelissaABond.com.